"*The Emotionally Exhausted Woman* is an invitation for women to re-imagine the inner work of self-care as a path of sacred presence. Full of wisdom and inspiration, we are reminded of the creativity, vitality, intelligence, and compassion that are always here/now, expressing the essence of who we are."

—**Tara Brach**, author of *Trusting the Gold*
and *Radical Acceptance*

"Don't be fooled by the size of this slim book. In just 147 mighty pages, Nancy Colier uses her insights as a psychotherapist to shake the comfortable box you live in and expose the roots of your depletion. She teaches you how to finally hang up your 'Good Girl' shoes, proudly own your needs, and mine your inner self for the restorative process you need."

—**Lesley Jane Seymour**, founder of www.coveyclub.com
and the *Reinvent Yourself with Lesley Jane Seymour* podcast,
and former editor in chief of *Marie Claire* and *More* magazines

"'Who is taking care of you?' is the first line in *The Emotionally Exhausted Woman*, and with that Nancy Colier takes us on a journey of self-discovery. Once we look inside and feel our feelings, and most of all speak up for ourselves, we can find our true and honest life. A book to savor!"

—**Sharon Salzberg**, author of *Lovingkindness*
and *Real Happiness*

"There isn't a woman alive who can't relate to this, nodding in agreement and desirous of a better way. Therapist and spiritual teacher Nancy Colier's latest book, *The Emotionally Exhausted Woman*, is like salve for the soul of the overly exhausted, overly worked, overly stressed modern woman caught in the spin cycle of busyness and bypassing. Beyond bubble baths and green juices, she imparts sage wisdom, insights, and tactical strategies that can be implemented so one can go from depleted to vital and empowered—body, mind, and spirit. It is an invitation to exhale and connect to our best selves in a healing and impactful way. Take her hand."

—**Kristen Noel**, editor in chief of *Best Self Magazine*

"This book will change how you live! If you're exhausted from taking care of everyone else's needs; depleted from feeling like you always having to be likable; if you've lost touch with what you really want and need. With compassion, insight, and humor, Nancy Colier empowers us to stand in our own shoes, take care of ourselves from the inside out, and live an authentic and truthful life."

—**Agapi Stassinopoulos**, author of *Speaking with Spirit*

"Nancy Colier spoke to all of us women, who were not given the tools and yet given a message that unless we are exhausted beyond repair, we are not doing enough. This book is a game changer for me and for generations to come. A reminder that we are inherently worthy of rest, love, and self-care. A reminder that I am not my productivity."

—**Tabitha Mpamira**, founder of Mutera Global Healing

"Truly inspirational. Colier invites us to be fully present, to nurture our deepest selves, and to replace being liked with being truthful as the highest form of self-care."

—**Daniela Ligiero, PhD**, CEO of Together for Girls, and cofounder of the Brave Movement

The
EMOTIONALLY EXHAUSTED WOMAN

WHY YOU'RE FEELING DEPLETED & HOW TO GET WHAT YOU NEED

NANCY COLIER

New Harbinger Publications, Inc.

Publisher's Note

NEW HARBINGER PUBLICATIONS is a registered trademark of New Harbinger Publications, Inc.

New Harbinger Publications is an employee-owned company.

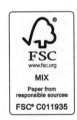

Copyright © 2022 by Nancy Colier
New Harbinger Publications, Inc.
5674 Shattuck Avenue
Oakland, CA 94609
www.newharbinger.com

All Rights Reserved

Cover design by Sara Christian

Acquired by Elizabeth Hollis Hansen

Edited by Teja Watson

Library of Congress Cataloging-in-Publication Data on file

Printed in the United States of America

24   23   22

10   9   8   7   6   5   4   3   2   1   First Printing

For Juliet, Gretchen, and Frederic

CONTENTS

WHO'S TAKING CARE OF YOU?

"Who's taking care of you?" This one question brings more women to tears than any other question I ask. After the tears, the response that comes is usually a simple *no one.*

Do you ever feel that no one is taking care of you, and perhaps more importantly, that you are also not caring for yourself—not in a way that's working? Women from every social, economic, educational, and racial background describe the same condition. "It's like having an umbilical cord attached to me, but it only flows one way—out." We spend our lives taking care of everyone's needs, playing our roles as caretakers of the world, being *good girls,* and working on self-improvement, but often at the expense of our own needs being met.

Have you always shown up for everyone in your life, anticipated and filled their needs, carried the emotional load, given everything you have emotionally, physically, and spiritually—given down to your bone marrow—and in the process, abandoned your own needs and turned away from something authentic and vital in you? Are you living in a way that's geared, above all else, to being liked? A way of being, essentially, that's missing *you* and what *you* need to be the truest expression of yourself.

It can take a long time to become aware of emotional exhaustion, and by the time you do, you may have developed a host of strategies for coping with it or anesthetizing yourself so you don't have to feel it. You may have even accepted at some level that your needs are not going to be met and you're not going to get to be *you* in any satisfying way, and that maybe that's just the way it is.

So, what are these needs that are not being met; what are we not getting that's resulting in our chronic exhaustion? While every woman has different desires and yearnings, there are certain needs that, when unrealized, create the emotional exhaustion and disconnection from self that's the normal state for so many of us.

As human beings, regardless of gender or identity, we share a longing to feel seen and known. And more specifically, to be seen and known *not* just for what we do and provide for others, but for who we genuinely *are*. We share a desire to live authentically, to be *real*, such that our outer experience is in alignment with our inner experience—to live a life that feels like *our* life, a life in which our truth is included.

Finally, and maybe most universally, we all yearn to feel loved and accepted—without criticism and judgment—which is the essence of feeling truly taken care of. We long for this connection not just from others, but from ourselves. If these needs are not met, or not met well enough, we end up in a state of depletion. As you embark on this journey, take a moment to ask yourself what kind of longing, absence, drive, experience, or burnout has brought *you* to this book? What hunger is going unfed in you?

Sometimes your emotional exhaustion feels unavoidable and acute. But it can also show up as a kind of wallpaper feeling, a background sense of dissatisfaction and incompleteness—an emptiness. You might have a hard time formulating the language to describe your exhaustion, and yet you feel it nonetheless.

What physical exhaustion is to the body, emotional exhaustion is to the heart and spirit. The condition manifests in many different forms: depression, anxiety, frustration, hopelessness, anger, fatigue, addiction, headaches, chronic pain, and insomnia…any and all can be manifestations of emotional exhaustion. In order to replenish ourselves and reconnect with our fundamental vitality, we must first understand the cause of our depletion. We can't fix something until we know what's broken—can't discover our real strength until we can see what's getting in its way.

This book was born from my curiosity and concern. After countless interviews with women, as well as decades of work with women clients in therapy, I was left wondering: Why do so many women describe themselves as emotionally exhausted? Why do so many of us experience ourselves as people-pleasing shells of something we used to be, or never were but maybe could be? Why do so many of us feel cut off from what we really need—and who we really are—untethered from some deeper well of nourishment? And, more important than all the whys, what can we do about it—how can we rediscover ourselves and reignite our internal vitality?

The cultural narrative goes like this: we are worthy, our needs are valid, and we have every right to express our truth. On a superficial level, the idea of authenticity is applauded in our society. *Be bold—be who you are. You be you!* We are encouraged to celebrate our uniqueness, voice our truth, and be…us. That's what's happening on the surface, but at a deeper level, such a way of living sits contrary to everything *else* we've been taught and been taught to be.

In reality, society's persistent dismissing and disparaging of women's needs, making fun of and negatively labeling women who openly express needs, idealizing women who appear need-less and self-sacrificing, has led us to create a relationship with our own needs that, like the one modeled, is critical and rejecting. Stop for a moment and think about your own life: consider the ways that your truth has been dismissed by others, and how you too may have participated in your own dismissal.

Despite all the progress we've made in the workforce, on the family and social front, the political stage, and everywhere else, so many women still believe that they're not supposed to have needs. Little ones maybe, here and there, but *not* the real ones we actually have, and not the inconvenient ones. Needs are still seen as a failing, and like most everything else, *our* failing.

This book is designed to help you become aware of your needs, and maybe more importantly, your *relationship* with your needs. To show you how to take care of yourself from the inside out, and not just play the part of someone who practices proper self-care. It's a guide for creating an internal state of vitality and authenticity that doesn't rely on finding the right partner, self-improvement plan, or facial cream. My goal is to shift your focus from taking care of everyone else to taking care of you, but in a brand-new way (which doesn't mean *not* taking care of others).

What's to come is a radically different approach to self-care—not the kind of temporary-fix, feel-good sort our current self-care industry promises, the kind that ultimately fails you. I offer something deeper, more reliable, and, I believe, infinitely more potent. One warning, however: If you decide to go on this journey, be ready to meet yourself, to unearth the *you* that's hiding under all the roles you play; be prepared to see the *you* that's free from all your pleasing adaptations. Be prepared to change.

My intention is to empower and encourage you to be more than just pleasing, more than just the parts you play for others. To dare you not just to know, but to speak and live from your actual truth. To help you discover who you actually are—beyond your ability to be likable. Ultimately, this book is about becoming a woman for whom it's more important to like herself than to be liked. If that sounds like what you want and need, and if you're willing to commit to this process, a time will come when you will trust your own knowing and stand firmly in your own shoes.

At its heart, this reading journey is about awareness. Through your investigation, you'll come to see the *truths* you've assumed about being a woman, the core beliefs you've been holding about your own needs, and the conditioning you've undergone, from society, family, education, media, and everywhere else—conditioning that's made you seek acceptance over authenticity. You'll become aware of your training to care for and manage others' needs at the expense of your own—to disappear to yourself so as to appear attractive to others.

Keep in mind, just by bringing light to your shadows, recognizing what's going on inside you, absorbing the message of this book, you are already doing the work. You are already changing.

Going forward, I describe what emotional exhaustion feels like and also what creates it. I throw open the door to *the likability cage:* the trap of always trying to be (and feeling like we have to be) pleasing in order to be emotionally safe—not judged and not rejected. I examine the individual bars that make up our cage, and the behaviors we assume to keep ourselves inside it and keep ourselves likable. All the ways we abandon ourselves while imagining we are taking care of ourselves.

I will lead us through the perilous and painful minefield of judgments, criticisms, and labels that our culture imposes on women (and we impose on ourselves) from *difficult* to *high maintenance* to *control freak*...the whole arsenal of threats that keep us silent and our needs in check. I look at early family environments—how your caretakers responded to your needs and how that shaped and distorted your own beliefs—as well as your strategies for trying to get your needs met.

Along the way, I unpack core beliefs—those imagined truths and assumed realities lingering in the shadows of our mind, which ultimately shape and guide our behavior. Core beliefs that kick up guilt, shame, and judgment, and if they stay in the shadows, continue getting in the way of what we need.

From there, we take a deep dive into the $11 billion self-care industry, the system that ultimately fails to address or remedy the real cause of our exhaustion.

And do I offer a solution? you're probably asking. Yes. A fundamentally different approach to taking care of yourself—practical, boots-on-the-ground tools for living a self-caring life, for being *you* in the world. A way of relating with the purpose of telling your truth rather than ensuring your likability. This book is a guide for how to live as a woman who knows that her experience matters and that *she* matters; a woman who respects and attends to her own needs, and who trusts her own knowing. A woman who is unshakably on her own side.

If you're still reading, my guess is that you identify with the feeling of emotional exhaustion, of not attending to yourself in a meaningful way, not getting your needs met, or perhaps not knowing what your needs even are. Or maybe the hope and possibility of a more truthful and vital life has kept your attention. Either way, it's good news that you're still here.

It's easy to talk about it, but *living* as a confident and truthful woman, who also has needs, is not easy. In fact, it can be downright risky. We face serious judgments for being who we really are…from men and women (ourselves included). Our conditioning has taught us to make sure that no one is ever displeased, which often doesn't line up well with being strong, visible, and genuinely honest. Tucking away our needs and our experience and focusing on making other people happy can seem like the safer and wiser choice.

But here's the thing: You don't have to abandon the people you love to take care of yourself. You also don't have to abandon yourself to be safe and happy. Over the years, I've accompanied innumerable women, a lot of them probably like you, on what I believe is the most important journey any of us ever take: from being whom you think everyone wants you to be...to being who you actually are. It's a process of relocating your center of gravity and North Star from the outside world to inside yourself. It's a homecoming.

No matter how many times I see a woman undergo this transformation—find her real voice, real needs, real strength, and real self, always in her unique style—I, too, am transformed. It's like watching a miracle every time. The sense of awe I carry for this process is ultimately why I wrote this book.

I invite you to read these pages slowly and carefully. Consider what it's like for *you* to be a woman in this society, the challenges you've personally faced, both internally and externally. Examine the ways you've been shaped—trapped or limited by your female conditioning. Pay close attention to how you relate to your own needs and how you allow (or don't allow) your needs to matter. You may find yourself asking, "But what do I *do*? What does it look like or feel like to do this work? Where do I begin?" The answer is simply to absorb the material, allow it into your consciousness, and let it work its way into your experience in whatever way it needs to.

We can and must look at this together to effect change. I encourage gathering with others along the way to bring this awareness to a personal and cultural level. To that end, I created a reading group guide that you can find at http://www.newharbinger.com/50157.

If you decide to embark on this journey, I would ask one favor: Promise me that you won't hold yourself to blame for what you discover along the way, that you will stay on your own side throughout this process. Let the words on these pages mean whatever they mean for you. There's no right way to experience them. But *do* experience them; don't turn this process into just another idea, another interesting addition to your self-care to-do list.

Keep it real and apply it in your own life (even if you never tell anyone that you're doing it). Use what works and leave the rest behind; not all of it will resonate, because you're *you* and not anyone else, and have lived your own unique road to here. Consider the reading of this book as a practice, one of listening deeply to your own experience and honoring *whatever* truth is uncovered.

1

WHERE DID WE GO?
THE LIKABILITY CAGE

"Miranda is an intelligent, engaging, and exceedingly likable woman. But even with all her likability, an aroma of exhaustion, even confinement, is evident in her presence. She appears like a golden bird inside a gilded cage." That was the note I wrote for myself after Miranda, whom I never forgot, left my office for the first time.

This forty-six-year-old, articulate, charismatic, professionally successful, stylish mother of two desperately wanted help creating a bolder and more authentic life. But here's where it got really interesting: she wanted that bolder and more authentic life *even* if it meant giving up "the benefits and rewards of being so *dependably pleasing*." While I didn't know it at the time, that one phrase was the seed of what would later become this book.

Miranda was a devoted mother to her children, a loving and attentive partner to her husband, a dedicated lawyer to her firm, a supportive daughter to her aging parents, a loyal friend to so many—what you might call an ideal modern woman. But in becoming all those things *to* all those people, she'd lost touch with her own wants and needs, who she needed to be—*to* (and for) herself. Her own longings, as they existed separately from all the people she served, had gone missing.

From the outside, Miranda was living the life we're supposed to want. She'd achieved and become everything our society tells us we should achieve and become. But on the inside, she felt cut off from something essential in her core—what she called her "*real* self." She felt untethered from her true vitality and power. Now, bone-tired from becoming and pleasing, she wanted instructions for unbecoming, and a road map for the return journey home to herself. She wanted to plug into something she could only describe as "me."

But Miranda had also spent her life cultivating the skill of being likable; she was afraid of needing what she needed and wary of the consequences for giving up her likability, which she imagined would be the loss of everything that mattered to her: her marriage, career, friends, and even her identity as a wonderful mother. The potential of *not* being pleasing felt threatening and unwise. She stated in no uncertain terms that she didn't want me to turn her into "a lady who lived with cats… entirely self-sufficient and alone, a woman who belonged to no one." Miranda was emotionally exhausted and unfulfilled, but also highly skeptical that any kind of better life, or even life worth living, existed if she wasn't *dependably pleasing.*

The Likability Cage

Belonging is a primal human need, because it's linked to our survival. Belonging to the herd means we won't be left behind, left unprotected, to die. But belonging is not just about being safe from physical harm, it's also about being safe from emotional harm—accepted, valued, and loved. We need to belong in order to feel emotionally and psychologically intact. Even though we're not living in the forest anymore and don't need the herd to protect us from being eaten, our need to belong still sits at the heart of everything we do. It still drives us.

But here's where it gets tricky: As women, we learn that the best way to belong, and thus survive, is to make ourselves pleasing, to be what other people want us to be. Likability then becomes our driving force and the operating system running below everything we do. Being liked means being included—wanted. And yet, this drive and pressure to be likable, while useful and protective in many ways, also becomes our cage. We start managing and controlling our behavior, accommodating, adjusting our wants and needs, and adapting our personality—in an effort to be pleasing, which then becomes who we think we are.

The Old Story

It's challenging to unearth the roots of women's exhaustion. When we approach the topic, we end up falling into our clichéd ideas about women who do too much. We jump to visions of the type-A, ultra-competent superwoman—the dynamo in the boardroom, bedroom, kitchen, and PTA. We envision that woman who can't say *no,* and who asks for (and receives) nothing for herself. Because we've internalized these stereotypes, when we hear about women who feel depleted, we slide into the habit of holding women responsible for, among other things, failing to properly take care of themselves. The overarching message, once again, is that if you're not getting what you need, it's probably your fault. When investigating your own exhaustion, I urge you *not* to fall into this trap. Your exhaustion is not your fault—even if you are a superwoman.

These well-worn clichés and narratives about women who do too much, coupled with the layers of complexity contained in this issue, make it a difficult one to unpack. It's no small task to freshly investigate your needs as a woman, honestly unravel the roots of your emotional exhaustion, and understand what makes it so chronic. It's equally challenging to come up with new and elevated solutions for the depletion that may be your current state. It can feel far easier to revert to the current crop of easy fixes, buying that shearling throw pillow or taking a sound bath, rather than investigating what's really unfed in you.

In truth, the odds have always been stacked against us women when it comes to getting our needs met, or taking care of our own needs, for that matter. The problem, which I address more deeply in later chapters, is that the very idea and practice of taking care of ourselves runs contrary to our most powerful conditioning: namely, to be selfless and self-sacrificing. It flies in the face of the more pervasive messaging that continually reminds us that we shouldn't need anything for ourselves. This chasm between who we're supposed to be and who we are—between what we *should* need and what we *do* need—sits at the heart of our emotional exhaustion.

The Perfect Woman

When I was a teenager, my uncle told me a story that raised questions that never fully left me. The story was about a man my uncle had known for many years, and also about the man's wife. Apparently, this man ventured out on most evenings; he could be found in the local pubs with friends, drinking buddies, and women…lots of women. Occasionally, he would check in with his wife from wherever he happened to be drinking, presumably to inform her of his whereabouts. When he did call, his wife always repeated the same words, which was the point of my uncle's story: "*Whenever* you get here, I'll be waiting for you." I remember clearly how the men in my family reacted, how they *ooh*ed and *aah*ed about his wife's response. "Wow," said one, "where can I buy that perfect woman?" while another asked if she had a sister.

Despite all of our progress as a society, there remains a strong and pervasive idea of the *perfect woman*. What's your picture of her? Is she strong, beautiful, smart, fit, helpful, confident, generous, loving, kind, forgiving, self-sacrificing? Does she fill everyone's needs but need nothing for herself? What does she offer that makes her so special and desirable? Thankfully, this perfect-woman image is changing with expanding gender identities, lifestyles, career paths, body types, and overall ways of being a woman in the world. And yet the perfect-woman image remains an ideal, a model for female-ness, and a strong *should* in our female psyche.

Ask yourself, *When you're not able to be this perfect imaginary woman, do you still believe that you should be her? Do you get frustrated with yourself because you can't meet this standard?* Our internal critic is often the voice of that *should*, the *shamer* and *blamer* that criticizes us for falling short of this female ideal. In striving to be the perfect woman, we are striving to be what we think will make us more desirable, more aligned with what's wanted. But in doing so, and judging ourselves for not being the fantasy, we're actually strengthening the bars of our cage.

Always and Forever Available

We learn a lot of things when we're young, often from watching our mothers and other women. We learn that being perfect means being available—*always* available to other people's needs. Being willing to move our own needs to the back burner when others' needs appear. Ask yourself: *If a friend, relative, coworker, or even stranger is in need, are you inclined to drop whatever you're doing to help out? Is saying "no" an unspoken taboo in your inner world?*

In my uncle's story, part of what made the man's wife so perfect—a woman men wanted to *buy*—was the fact that she was always available to her man. She was waiting at home to receive him with love and without questions, needs, or expectations...available to serve him when *he* needed it. But holding ourselves to a standard of unrelenting availability, while it may make us more popular and desirable, ultimately reinforces the belief that we are valuable *because* of our availability; we are liked *because* we put others first, which then keeps us enslaved to the same behavior and the same exhaustion.

Hypervigilance to What Other People Think (of Us)

In order to stay likable, we've learned to stay vigilantly attuned not just to other people's needs, but to what other people think of us. Consider your own experience: Are you hyper-focused on other people's perceptions of you? Do you trust (and prioritize) their perceptions over your own, throw out your own knowing in favor of their opinions of you?

It's logical, in some sense, to focus on getting other people to like us; if we're successful at it, chances are we won't be rejected or abandoned. But in focusing our attention and energy on what other people think of us (or what we think they think), we end up farming out our self-esteem and self-experience, our very identity, to family, friends, partners, experts, and whomever else we think might know us better than we know ourselves. We hand over our most intimate and essential questions: *What's my truth? What do I want and need? What makes me like myself? Who do I think I am?* These are then replaced by *Who do you think I am? How do you think I'm doing? What do you need me to need?* and *Who do I need to be so that you will like me?*

When it comes to the answers to life's most important questions, we've learned to trust others in place of ourselves. Consequently, we never become the ones who know better, never become the authority in our own lives.

Dismissing Ourselves

With our attention focused on others' needs and perceptions, and naturally, on satisfying those needs and shaping those perceptions, we quickly learn to distrust and dismiss our own experience. We disregard our own knowing, imagining it's wiser to stop listening to our truth, and reject ourselves as a source of wisdom. Eventually, we stop believing that we *can* be trusted to determine what's best for us and even to determine our own truth. As we imagine it, if we really stood in our own shoes and let our own experience guide us, we would lose what matters to us.

And so, we hand our truth off to others to decide, and ironically, are rewarded for it. Our doubting ourselves becomes evidence of our flexibility and cooperativeness, which then becomes another way to ensure our belonging. Our own experience is best decided by others, which in its own strange way keeps us likable.

By the time we've become women, we're highly adept at ignoring and invalidating our own voice, the voice inside us that knows what's true for us and knows what we want and need—if we were to listen. By now, that voice may be whispering in your ear, and maybe even (if you're lucky) shouting for your attention.

What We Need Is Out There

Further contributing to our likability cage is the belief that what we need lies somewhere outside of us...if only we could find it. Many of us spend our entire lives seeking this something or someone that will fulfill us and reunite us with ourselves. We go searching for the key to the castle, to the self-help experts, our partners, people that know us, the media, celebrities—convinced that what we need is somewhere else. But we don't stop to consider that maybe the key is in our own pocket.

Staying Silent

When I was listening to my uncle's story of the perfect woman, I remember feeling both confusion and dismay at what was being celebrated by these men I loved and trusted. What's remarkable, however, is that even at that tender age, I already understood that if I were to speak up and make my feelings heard, show my discontent, I would have been dismissed as one of those overly dramatic and hormonal young women. While I probably couldn't have articulated it, I understood at a visceral level that speaking my actual truth would have posed a serious threat to being included and adored...a risk I wasn't willing to take.

One of our most ingrained and habitual behaviors is that of staying silent and *not* speaking our mind. We harbor a deep belief that it's self-protective to keep our real feelings to ourselves, particularly when they conflict with other people's feelings. We're convinced that our silence and agreeableness improves our chances of being liked, which it probably does. In order to avoid being negatively judged, we make the choice again and again to *not* say what we really think and feel, to shape-shift our real truth into something pleasant and nice, and adjust our experience so that it works for everyone. Maybe you've told yourself it's a fair trade: you give up your voice, truth, integrity, and the chance to be truly known, but in exchange, you get to be appreciated and wanted. You get to fit in. Agreeableness and silence then win the day as the more trustworthy ways to take care of yourself, and thus become your strategy of choice.

Being Invisible

It's confusing, really: the message we get from so many sources is that we should ask for what we need, be authentic, and practice self-care, but at the same time, we're mightily rewarded for being accommodating, making other people happy, and being selfless. If you look closely, the self-care we're encouraged to practice is in fact for a selfless self. Such is the female quandary.

Furthermore, because we believe that our selflessness is respected and desired, we expect it of ourselves. The more we insist on not having needs, the harder it is to ask for what we need, and consequently, to get our needs met. The more we require ourselves to be selfless, the more we strengthen the system that rewards our selflessness. And round and round we go…away.

Valued for Giving

From the time we can hold up our little girl head, that head starts getting filled up with ideas about what it means to be a *good girl*. Specifically, we learn that being a *good girl* means being giving and helpful. The more we give, the more we're complimented and respected—cherished. Not surprisingly, this then becomes the way we determine our own value; we feel worthy for being giving, and expect ourselves to give—so as to earn our worthiness. The result is that we give until we have nothing left to give, imagining that our giving is also our getting. But in doing so, we trap ourselves in a way of living that keeps us perpetually focused on other people's needs and how we can satisfy them, imagining that we'll get our needs met through taking care of others. A way of living that ultimately depletes us. In the process, we once again fortify the very system that exhausts us.

Blaming Ourselves for Our Needs

Finally, there's one other behavior worth mentioning here, so deeply ingrained in us as to make it tough to recognize. The behavior is this: We blame ourselves for our own needs. More specifically, for having the wrong needs, being undeserving of our needs, and of course, not being able to make our needs disappear.

The real dilemma is that we've been taught to relate to our own needs as a problem; our needs are something we're doing wrong, and more treacherously, something that makes *us* wrong. Our needs are not just unwanted and unwelcome, but also threatening to our self-esteem—and, it goes without saying, to our likability.

As with all of our adaptive behaviors, we blame ourselves, paradoxically, in an effort to improve our chances of being accepted and, therefore, safe. But with this particular adaptation, we simultaneously eliminate any hope of building a healthy relationship with our needs and with ourselves. Since we are to blame for the problem that is our needs, since we are the problem itself, the possibility of ever being willing to take care of ourselves—or even *like* ourselves, a prerequisite—is, well...impossible.

So, returning to our question: Why are so many women emotionally exhausted? And furthermore, why do we assume that feeling exhausted is just the way life is? If you think about it, how could it be any other way when our primary job in life is to be liked? And when we believe that ensuring our likability *is* taking care of ourselves and is our best shot at being happy. But perhaps most insidiously, when we believe that being likable requires us to attend to others' needs over our own, silence our inner and outer voices, and distrust our own knowing. In short, abandoning ourselves. If we believe all of this, which many of us do, why then would we attend to our own needs? For what purpose? And how would we go about caring for and about ourselves without giving up everything else we need?

In the next chapter, I will look more closely at the specific messages we receive and internalize as women, and particularly those that keep us trapped and exhausted.

2

CULTURE: ENFORCING THE WOMAN NOT TO BE

What does it mean to be female? It's a question that our patriarchal culture sets out to answer for us—what we should look like, need, want, think; how we should behave, and the space we're allowed to occupy—without consequences to our belonging and likability. Ultimately, we're taught how to be female.

But any time we're learning how to be, we're also learning how *not* to be, which often is the stronger message and the one that really sticks. While there's no official *dos* and *don'ts* list, nevertheless, as girls and women, we come to understand quickly and clearly who we're *not* supposed to be and what will cost us our belonging and approval.

One caveat, however: While I describe a society that's patriarchal by nature and a number of my examples include men who appear to be on the wrong side of the story, men are not to blame for women's emotional exhaustion. In fact, men are also caught in our current system, which encourages women to be selfless and pleasing and judges us for having needs. Awareness of the female experience and the societal cage in which women live can also liberate men in their relationships, as well as enhance the possibilities for all male-female relating.

The purpose of becoming aware of these hidden and not-so-hidden messages is so that we can stop being controlled by them. We bring these messages to light so as to disempower them—so they no longer dictate our behavior. Once you can see what you're believing, what you're afraid of and why, and furthermore, how you're accommodating and controlling yourself to allay these fears, maintain likability, and ultimately, escape judgment, you can then break free from the system. With greater awareness, and without these fears blocking you, you can stop living defensively and become more than just well behaved. You can live spontaneously, without always having to police your needs and manage yourself; you can live as who you *are* rather than who you *should* and *shouldn't* be.

What follows are some of the judgments and labels we face and navigate on a daily basis as females, and indeed that we may accept as just part of being a woman in this culture.

"You're So Difficult"

It's a powerful word, *difficult,* and one that packs a lot of punch when used as a criticism against us. *Difficult* is one of those judgments that's frequently put on women whose needs are *too* visible. And so, we'll start with what we know as the *difficult woman.*

Chloe was in a fresh relationship and over the moon about her new guy. She and her boyfriend had been together for three wonderful months when he invited her to accompany him on a day trip to the beach. Now, Chloe was not a beach person; she actually didn't like the beach. But when it came to a day with her new boyfriend, her dislike of the sun and countless bad experiences with severe sunburns on her fair skin all went out the window. She was thrilled to spend the day with her new man.

Unfortunately, when they arrived and began setting up their blankets on the sand, Chloe realized that the bottle of sunscreen in her bag was empty. Her boyfriend was a beach bum; he didn't think about sunscreen and certainly hadn't brought any. Chloe could feel her anxiety spiking: she was facing at least six hours in the direct sun, with no shade to be found.

Chloe then excused herself, she said, to grab a bottle of water from the snack stand, but they didn't sell sunscreen at the shop, and so she returned with two waters and without what she really needed. She knew that the local town was only about a mile away, but it would mean dragging their cooler, blanket, and the whole setup back to the car, driving into town, and then coming back and starting again. It felt like more effort than her need (and she) deserved. So she decided to tough it out.

She spent the day feeling anxious about the sunburn she could already feel happening, but at the same time, paralyzed by the fear of being seen as a woman who was *difficult*. After her boyfriend dropped her off that night, she took herself to urgent care as she was dangerously near heat stroke (none of which she shared with him). Sadly, the choice to *not* be seen as a bother resulted in severe sun poisoning, a missed day of work, and a body covered in blisters.

Chloe didn't want to be one of those "difficult divas who always has special requests." She didn't want to have a problem or be a problem. What she wanted, more than anything, was for her boyfriend to like her—which in her mind meant being the *chill girlfriend* who needed nothing and had no issues. She was convinced that these were the traits of a woman who was desirable.

A woman's ability to be accommodating and easygoing, which is code for *without needs,* is a big selling point in a woman's attractiveness quotient in this culture. As one man put it, somewhat joking, and somewhat not, "The less of a pain in the ass a woman is, the more appealing." A woman is deemed difficult when her needs require effort or a change in behavior from anyone else or when she can't take care of her needs quietly and on her own. So too, she's considered difficult when what she needs is different from what someone else thinks she should need—or maybe more accurately, what someone else needs her to need.

"How Dare You Be So Selfish!"

"But isn't it selfish for me to want to spend time alone? Doesn't that make me a bad mother?" Anne was pained and conflicted about needing time for herself. "Just an hour or two on the weekends is all I really need. But that's not fair to my kids; shouldn't I be willing to put their needs first? It's so selfish, isn't it...to put myself ahead of them."

And there it is in a nutshell: To give ourselves what we need, even for just an hour, is an act of selfishness. Self-caring becomes *selfish* and time for ourselves is time *taken away* from others. Attending to our own needs, in whatever small way, makes us someone who does whatever she wants and thinks of *only* herself.

The reality is, from the time we're born, we're praised and admired for putting other people ahead of ourselves. "Look how beautifully she gives her toys away, such a good sharer!" "What a sweet girl...see how she takes the smaller cookie and lets her brother have the big one?" The message is uncomplicated and direct—you're good because you put others ahead of you. The message's more subtle counterpart: other people's getting what they want is more important than your getting what you want. And even more subtle than that: other people's getting what they want *is* what you want. Having learned that our value is derived from how much we give to others, it follows then that being called selfish is the worst possible criticism, as it brings our basic worth into question.

Maddie, a dear friend, had never ordered a meal when we went out to dinner with her family. After many years of noticing this, I finally asked her why she never got her own food. Her answer, which came effortlessly, was that she was just so busy getting her kids fed that she didn't have time to feed herself. But more importantly, that she derived so much pleasure and satisfaction from watching her two boys enjoy their food that she didn't need to eat. Their joy was her joy, and nourishment enough; their needs met were her needs met.

It's no wonder that we are the caretakers of the world: the nurses, social workers, teachers—the helpers. Supposedly, it's not just our worth, but also our happiness that's to be derived from making other people happy. We should be fulfilled through the process of giving, knowing that we are successfully satisfying our most important responsibility as women.

When we acknowledge our own needs, and maybe even treat them like they matter, we're immediately hit with the fear and very real threat of being judged as selfish. But before anyone else can do it, we usually do it to ourselves; *selfish* is often the first line of attack our inner critic uses against us. It's a condemnation I hear every day in my office—most often, I'm sad to say, by women against themselves.

The fear of being selfish is coded into our early programming, the belief that taking care of our own needs is self-serving, self-centered, self-indulgent, and just way too much *self*. At the same time, considering our own needs implies discounting everyone else's needs. If we care about ourselves then we don't care about others; it's *either/or*. When we only have two options—selfless or selfish—the choice is obvious.

"You're Such a Control Freak"

Rada was carrying a heavy heart; her youngest daughter would soon be leaving for college; she was suffering and needed to talk about it with her husband. Because he was easily distracted, the car seemed like a good place to share what she was feeling. She hoped that she could talk about her grief and anxiety, and also that they could discuss their own relationship and her fear that there wouldn't be enough glue to hold them together in an empty nest. Rada needed reassurance and, really, just to be heard.

After a few minutes of sharing, her husband started happily humming to a song on the radio and dancing in his seat. Rada gently told him that it felt odd and maybe a little tone-deaf that he would be dancing and singing at this moment when she was sad and sharing something so important to her. Rada then kindly asked her husband if he could refrain from dancing and singing; if he could just listen or maybe engage in some way with what she was feeling. He said nothing and then offered an agitated, "I'm listening." He seemed then, as Rada put it, "like a grenade with its pin about to be pulled."

And so, too hurt to continue, Rada stopped speaking mid-sentence and got quiet. After a couple minutes, she broke the silence: "Why do my feelings make you so angry? All I need to hear is that we'll figure it out, we'll change, we'll find a new way to be a couple. All I need is a little reassurance, for you to *be* with me in this…it's not often but yes, every blue moon, I ask you, my husband, for some kindness. Is that too much?"

With those words, the pin was pulled and the grenade erupted. After a few loud expletives, it went like this: "You are such a control freak…you control absolutely everything and everyone. Just write the script for me and I'll follow it; control everything I say and do, that's obviously what you want. Why don't you find yourself a robot you can program exactly to your liking, then maybe you can get what you need." After that, they both went silent.

As strange as this interaction may sound, I hear these sorts of exchanges all the time. Rada shared her experience and asked for what she needed, which was understanding and empathy. That honesty was then judged as her being controlling. And that was the end of Rada's getting anything close to what she needed. In fact, labeling a woman a *control freak* is a method of controlling her and shutting her up, which is usually exactly what it does.

Almost every day in my office, a woman recounts a story in which she is labeled *controlling*, or the term more frequently used, a *control freak*. Controlling is a judgment used against us when we do any number of things—but most often, when we ask that our needs be taken seriously and dare to request that someone change their behavior on account of us.

Of all the judgments we women face in coming out with our needs, being called controlling is one of the most powerful and effective ones for closing us down and forcing our needs back into hiding—convincing us that, no matter what it costs us, we must stop controlling others and start controlling *ourselves*. Why is this particular label so effective? Because we wholeheartedly believe it; we believe that we're a control freak when we ask another person to shift their behavior *because* of us—our needs or our feelings. For many women, to be perceived as controlling is so shameful and unattractive as to make us unwilling to risk it.

The label *controlling* is a criticism designed to make us feel bad about ourselves: ashamed and aggressive, overbearing and unfeminine, domineering and dominating, and really, just plain *gross*. And it works. At the same time, it makes us feel imprisoned, frustrated, and angry. This judgment, when believed, renders us powerless, with no options for expressing ourselves. The more we say, the more controlling we're accused of being. We're trapped. Ironically, calling a woman controlling turns out to be the most effective way of controlling her, and simultaneously, getting her to control herself.

"What Else Are You Going to Demand?"

While similar to *difficult*, the criticism *demanding*, when used against a woman, carries its own unique and damaging punch. When we're perceived as demanding, the insinuation is that we not only require too much, ask for more than we deserve, and need more than we should, but also that we feel entitled to all of that, which makes us even more unlikable.

My friend Ana recently asked her husband if he could run an errand for their son, drop something off for the boy at his school. Her husband responded with a sarcastic, "Anything else you might need, your majesty?" The implication in her husband's remark was that she was asking for more than she had the right to ask for (and need). It made Ana feel pushy, as if she had overstepped her rights and been caught mistakenly assuming she deserved anything. She felt "like one of those demanding, bossy women who go around brazenly assigning tasks and feeling entitled." I had to talk my friend out of the distorted, gas-lit pseudo-reality her husband had constructed (and she had internalized), to remind her of the ridiculousness of his implication.

Together, we did some reality-checking, remembering how small the task was that she had requested, how infrequently she asked for anything, and also the fact that the royal favor wasn't even for her, but rather for *their* child. She had every right to ask her husband to do something for the family, or her, without apology.

"You Don't Just Have Needs, You're Needy!"

The experience of having needs exists for every gender (as well as those who don't identify with gender). But for women specifically, our culture collapses the natural experience of having needs into the unappealing and dysfunctional state of being *needy*. When need becomes *needy*, it suggests that our needs are excessive, more than our fair share, and burdensome. And if our needs are burdensome, then *we* are burden-some. At the same time, the judgment of *needy* comes with the implica-tion that we are weak and overly dependent on others—helpless. When we add that one letter to the word *need*, two very different phenomena are conflated into one pathology. In the process, we turn our own needing, this sacred intuitive knowing in us, into something broken and shameful. We transform *need*, which arises from our deepest wisdom and most self-protective nature, and which is in fact needing on *our* behalf—pleading *our* case—into something damning and damaging to us.

Maria and her boyfriend had been dating for six months. They saw each other every weekend, but only occasionally during the work week. And yet, if Maria didn't contact Sam, the weekend would come and go without a plan and without their seeing each other. When she did reach out to him, he always seemed happy to hear from her; he was compli-mentary and affectionate when they were together, but still, would never initiate their dates.

Understandably, this caused Maria to feel insecure and guarded in the relationship. "If I stopped calling, would the relationship just disap-pear without a trace?" she wondered. And yet, despite her confusion and insecurity, she kept muddling along, making the relationship happen, making herself desirable, and keeping her mouth shut.

When I asked Maria the obvious question—why she didn't raise the issue with Sam—she said that she didn't want to be seen as needy. She understood, intellectually, how unacceptable the whole situation was and that she deserved better, but she was still too scared to bring it up. No matter how confused and rejected it made her feel, or how resentful she was becoming, still the risks outweighed the suffering. When I asked her what those risks were, specifically, she explained that she was afraid he would think she was one of those desperate women who always required reassurance, validation, and knowing where the relationship *stood.* (This last part was accompanied with air quotes and a crinkled-up face.)

Wanting to know why Sam had never invited her out on a date would have been letting the cat out of the bag—admitting that she did, in fact, have emotional needs. The big disappointment for Sam (or so she feared) would be that his girlfriend couldn't just roll with anything and wasn't okay with whatever worked for Sam. It would expose her need to know what was going on in the relationship, which would mean that she was, as she put it, "needy and pathetic."

"I've spent my life championing women's issues, blathering on about empowered women. How is it possible that I need a man to reassure me and tell me our relationship is secure? It's embarrassing." Maria's needs implied (to Maria) that she was one of those pathetic women who needed a man to be okay—a woman who couldn't be a real feminist and who obviously couldn't function on her own. In order to be perceived as strong and capable, and experience ourselves as such, we believe that we can't need anything from anyone.

"You're Impossible to Please...That's Why You're Unhappy"

While similar to both *difficult* and *demanding,* the label *impossible to please* has earned its own special place on the list of potential put-downs women navigate when expressing our needs.

Laura woke up on her birthday to find a beautifully wrapped present on the pillow next to her. She brought the gift into the living room and gave her partner a big hug. Inside the wrapping, Laura discovered a set of candlestick holders, obviously expensive. She thanked her partner profusely and told her how much she appreciated them, and her.

The next day in my office, Laura was crying about those same candlestick holders. The reality, under all her gratitude, was that her partner's gift made her feel unknown, *not* special. As she described, "I'm a woman with many interests and hobbies, none of which are candles. I don't even light candles on Hanukkah. It felt like my girlfriend went online, googled 'best birthday gifts for your woman,' and bought the first thing she saw. None of it had anything to do with me...it was just something that she could feel good about giving."

The impersonalness of her girlfriend's choice made Laura feel lonely and not known. But not surprisingly, Laura had absolutely no intention of sharing her feelings with her partner. "I wouldn't dare," she said, laughing. "If I did, I'd be left with those same damn candlesticks and a big sandwich board around my neck that said, 'Impossible to please.'" As Laura saw it, any conversation that suggested her partner's gift wasn't perfect, and that her efforts were anything other than deeply appreciated, would have immediately led to judgment—of Laura. She would be a problem and there would be something wrong with her response.

We fear being labeled as one of those women who's never satisfied—a woman for whom nothing is ever enough. Not being pleased makes *us* to blame for our disappointment, and so we suppress our experience, make others feel pleased, and behave as if we're satisfied.

"You're One of Those Angry Women"

And the list goes on... Women who are honest about what they need and not afraid when other people are uncomfortable—women for whom being liked is not the number-one concern—are not only branded as *difficult*, *demanding*, and *impossible to please*, but also *angry*, which goes hand in hand with its sister insults: *nasty* and *bitter*. Our society has made a mockery of the woman who asks that her needs be taken seriously; the woman who speaks her mind, sometimes even with intensity, is an object of contempt and ridicule in our society. These days, she's often called a *Karen*, regardless of how respectfully she behaves. This woman is dismissed as harsh, shrill, neurotic, and of course, the always looming badge of degradation, as a bitch. Truth be told, we (both men and women) take pleasure in hating this woman.

"Do You Have to Be So Aggressive?"

Karoline grew up in a traditional home; the women of the family were the caretakers and in charge of homemaking duties. Except for one: Aunt Nora. Successful in her career, attractive, fashionable, well-educated, and opinionated, Nora was a strong woman who kept up her end of the conversation. She did her fair share to help at meals, but she was more than just a helper. When the family was speaking kindly of her, she was known as "a powerhouse" and "a force to be reckoned with." When they weren't being kind, she was known as "the bulldozer," or simply "the bull."

But Karoline's parents complained vehemently about what they called "Nora's massive presence." *Who does she think she is?* her parents would regularly ask, disparagingly. The family narrative on Nora was that she *acted like a man*; she had *the balls* to ask for what she needed (and to even assume that she should get it).

But despite their negative spin, Karoline remembered liking and admiring her aunt because she was interesting, interested in Karoline, and fun to be around. Aunt Nora was the kind of woman who wasn't afraid to express what she thought and felt, the kind of woman Karoline thought was cool—an opinion that clearly no one else shared. And so, understandably, Karoline kept her feelings to herself.

Over time, under the tutelage of her parents' judgments and mockery, Karoline's admiration eventually waned. She became convinced that Nora was precisely the kind of woman *not* to become, the kind of woman that no man would ever want and no woman would ever trust or befriend.

So Karoline too learned to turn away—not just from her aunt, but from her own ideas, interests, and passions, and from those qualities in herself that she shared with her aunt. She learned to present herself as quieter, sweeter, and more vanilla than she felt, to tuck away her own wants and needs, so as not to risk being one of those women who demands to be seen, and is aggressively herself. Karoline's conditioning taught her that speaking up, having an opinion, and occupying a real seat at the table were ballsy and brash moves—antagonistic and confrontational. And they made other people uncomfortable—which led to rejection. The message was clear: a strong, present, and unapologetic woman was also an unattractive, unfeminine, and unlikable woman.

"There's Too Much—of You!"

Since I had known Vanessa, which was many years now, she had lived in fear of being seen and judged as *too much*. She, like Karoline, had spent her life trying not to be too big of a presence—too loud, too forceful, too visible—to take up too much space, physically, emotionally, intellectually, or in any other way.

Vanessa remembered her father using the term *leaker* for any woman who, in her words, "refused to protect others from her existence." When a woman showed up fully, without apologizing for her presence and without feeling ashamed of herself, Vanessa's father felt personally offended and even violated. He claimed that such a woman was broadcasting herself and unconsciously screaming, *See me!* Behind her back, he would judge her as an attention glutton and accuse her of being inappropriate and unable to contain herself—which, to Vanessa, meant being unwilling to make herself small, and therefore tolerable.

Not surprisingly, Vanessa's mother was soft-spoken, slim, "bordering on emaciated," and always amenable—a person who, in Vanessa's words, "had no opinions and seemed to take up no space at all...more like a gas than a solid." It was understandable—perhaps a survival mechanism or maybe why he chose her.

And in case the message wasn't clear enough, Vanessa's father would frequently remind his daughter that women who were *too much* were guilty of spewing their emotional muck on others. Women who were too *in your face* were repellent; according to her father, men worried that such women would *eat them alive*. As a result, the threat of being perceived as too much made Vanessa feel perpetually ashamed of her potential *too-muchness*. She felt, as she described it, "gross," as if her too-muchness was leaking out despite her strident efforts to contain it. She'd spent her life staying carefully bottled up and well managed, with her needs sealed inside an impenetrable vault—hidden from everyone, including herself.

The embarrassment and humiliation that comes with the label *too much* keeps us tightly restrained and vigilantly monitoring ourselves. The goal becomes to be smaller and quieter—*less* than we naturally are. We seek to become someone with whom others can always feel comfortable, who doesn't take up too much space or demand too much attention, and doesn't make others feel too small or swallowed up by our too-muchness. In so doing, we get to remain likable and beyond reproach.

"Aren't You Conceited!"

Clara was an A student in high school. She was the girl who always knew the answers to the teachers' questions. She was also a varsity athlete and an accomplished trumpet player. But though Clara had many talents and skills, she wasn't just gifted—she also worked hard at everything she did.

While Clara may sound incredibly lucky, in fact, possessing such gifts and talents, being good at so many things didn't make life easy for

her. She described that time in her life as "hard, confusing, and scary."
It was a time when Clara, like so many women, had a distinctly conflicted relationship with her own power and potential.

Years later, Clara still talked about how painful it was to keep her
hand down when she knew the answers and wanted to contribute. She
recalled keeping track of how many times each day she'd been called on
by the teacher, ever-careful not to let that number get too high—not to
shine as brightly or obviously as she was capable of shining. In one particularly embarrassing memory, she described pretending not to understand the material in class, even though she understood it perfectly. She
felt perpetually in danger of being seen as arrogant and better-than—
too full of herself.

Her desire to participate was far outweighed by her fear of being
seen as smart, powerful, and talented. For many women, such attributes
are experienced as a challenge and a liability. Powerful and smart
women are often judged as conceited, arrogant, and self-important. If
you're powerful and smart as a woman, the assumption is that you *think*
you're powerful and smart, and *that* is unacceptable.

The message we women receive is confusing: *Be smart, be confident,
be powerful, get noticed...but don't be too smart, too confident, too powerful, or get too noticed.* And definitely don't be too much smarter or too
much more confident or noticed than anyone else. Unfortunately, it's
never clear where the line is or what exactly is *too* much. We spend a lot
of energy worrying about how our abilities and talents will be perceived
and experienced by others. We feel it's our responsibility to make sure
that no one else feels inadequate, threatened, or less-than as a result of
our strengths (and hard work). We're allowed to be talented—to a
point—but not if our talent makes anyone else feel less talented, or
worse, untalented. At that point, our abilities become a problem, and
something we're perpetrating on someone else. Subsequently we're held
to blame for how other people feel about themselves—in relation to us.

Before we can fully own or actualize our power, or even feel comfortable with it, we must first make sure that other people are okay with it. The result is that we're left trying to walk an impossibly thin line: to be all that we are, celebrate our efforts, take pride in our abilities, and simultaneously, dodge the barrage of negative judgments and projections that our power triggers in others.

"Are You High-Maintenance or What?!"

No conversation on women and needs would be complete without everyone's favorite label: *high-maintenance*. Such is the popular term for the woman who orders her dressing on the side or wants anything other than the easiest choice. As one of those women who sometimes orders off the menu, the act of asking for what I want and saying no to what I don't want and didn't ask for—even after decades of talking about this issue—has never felt risk free or easy. While I don't allow myself to be shamed into silence and don't change course on account of the judgments and smirks I receive for my *special* requests, still, it's a challenging and stressful choice every time—to not abandon my own needs so that life can be just a little easier for everyone...myself included.

As women, we learn to apologize for wanting what we want in a thousand inventive and charming ways. In trying to get our needs met and still be liked, we make fun of ourselves and call ourselves every name in the book: *high-maintenance, neurotic, uptight, particular, rigid,* and of course, *crazy*. No matter how evolved we may be, still—when asking for what we want (or don't want) to eat, drink, or swallow, emotionally or physically—we feel shame, anxiety, frustration, and fear.

Recently I was out for breakfast with a friend. She ordered toast, "dry, with no butter." I heard her say those exact words, which she said very clearly and politely. But the waiter didn't write anything down on his pad when she said it. I thought about asking him if he had heard my friend, but refrained, practicing my own advice of *not* taking care of everyone else. When my friend's toast arrived, I wasn't surprised to see that it was buttered. She saw it too, but said nothing.

After a few minutes of watching her ignore her toast, I asked her why she didn't just send it back, since she had been very clear about wanting it dry. I think I already knew why not, but I wanted to hear it from her. She said, "Honestly, I just don't have the energy…I don't want to be that crazy, high-maintenance woman who is so demanding and impossible to satisfy. You know, the neurotic freak. I know I should fight the good fight, for all women, but I don't have it in me today." Her words, which I'd heard women say hundreds of times in hundreds of different ways, on this particular day, coming from my strong, smart, capable, and kind friend, made me deeply sad—for all of us. It also convinced me that I needed to keep writing this book.

While ordering off-the-menu is the most obvious form of what we mock as high-maintenance, in fact there are countless ways a woman can fall prey to this particular criticism. A woman who cares about or spends time on her physical appearance is deemed high-maintenance, as is one who wants something different from what she's supposed to want. Essentially, a woman who asks for what she wants and needs, and believes that those wants and needs are valid and that they matter—*she* has a bullseye on her forehead when it comes to this particular label.

Simply put, the label *high-maintenance* suggests that we require too much work to maintain, demand too much energy and effort (to keep happy), and ultimately, need more than we deserve. We're a problem… difficult, demanding, overbearing, controlling, neurotic, impossible to please, anal, tightly wrapped, unstable, anxious, type-A, obsessive, and probably crazy too. *High-maintenance* contains all the negative judgments, all rolled into one. No matter how evolved, self-confident, and aware we are, still, we have to face these condemnations when we request something that requires effort from another person—even if it's just writing down the word *dry*.

So, when that high-maintenance woman refuses to throw herself under the bus, to join the prevailing opinion that she's a pain in the ass and there's something wrong with her; when she finds the strength to stay on her own side, the courage to hold others accountable for acknowledging her needs; when she dares to behave as if her needs matter, regardless of how politely she does it, the criticisms quickly intensify. Soon, she's no longer just neurotic, controlling, and crazy, but now she's nasty, aggressive, belligerent, and hostile too. She's got the whole shaming and blaming arsenal headed her way.

The Need Police

For many women, expressing real needs is just not worth the risk of being ridiculed, shamed, blamed, dismissed, belittled, insulted, patholo-gized...and the list goes on. It's not worth being put in a box with all the other women who are *that*. No woman wants to be put in *that* box. And so, we learn to stay silent, ignore our own needs, or pretend that our needs are being taken care of when they're not. At the same time, we get really good at behaving as if we don't have any needs, and believing it too. All this to try and stay out of harm's way. And these coping strat-egies leave us feeling emotionally exhausted, inauthentic, and lonely. And worst of all, at war with our own needs.

In truth, we don't only fear being *seen* in all these negative ways, but we also fear actually possessing these negative qualities, *being* the unlik-able women such societal messages suggest. We view ourselves through the lens of the machine, internalize the criticisms, and absorb them into our self-image. The result is that we learn to feel like we're not enough, and guilty; we *are* the unlikable people we're accused of being. Consequently, our relationship with ourselves carries the same judg-mental and dismissive flavor that the relationship society has modeled for us.

The fact is, we approach our own needs with an attitude shaped not only by the cultural messaging machine, but also by the ways in which our needs were responded to by our primary caretakers. In the next chapter, I'll invite you to step back and explore your relationship with needs through the lens of your family. Specifically, the ways in which your childhood caretakers laid the ground for how you relate and respond to your needs now.

3

FAMILY: LEARNING TO NEED (AND NOT NEED)

This is a book about getting our needs met and meeting them for ourselves—as women. But before we can have an in-depth conversation about making that happen, we have to better understand our relationship with our own needs: how we think and feel about needs, why we respond to them in the ways we do, and why we are so distrusting and judgmental of our own experience. And ultimately, how we became such an inhospitable environment for our own truth.

So far, we've been investigating the conditioning that discourages us from having needs and the emotional dangers that result from expressing needs in our society. But in fully unpacking our conflicted and complicated relationship with needs, it behooves us to consider where it all began. And indeed, the attitude with which our childhood caretakers responded to our emotional needs is critically influential in shaping how we respond to our own needs as adults. Our caretakers were our original models: they taught us what our needs *do* to other people, and therefore, what they will *do* to us; they were our benchmark for how our needs impact our important relationships and basic emotional safety. At the same time, they also showed us what to believe and expect about the possibility of actually getting our needs met.

Your primary task and goal in childhood is to survive it intact, emotionally and physically, which can mean many different things depending on the level of awareness and empathy in your family. In an effort to achieve this goal, you figure out quickly whether it's safe to feel, reveal, or even *have* needs. You learn to manage your internal experience, so as to secure your safety and *not* end up unloved, and to maintain a good-enough self-image to be able to function in the world. Boiled down, your family teaches you whether your needs *matter*. And furthermore, whether *you* matter. Your current relationship with your own needs is, in large part, the result of this early education.

If you had caregivers who were emotionally available, able to listen and attend to you with kindness and meet your emotional needs enough of the time, it's likely that your attitude toward your own needs, to some degree, will also be empathic and supportive. Raised by caretakers who were sufficiently attuned and understanding of your needs, you are less likely to view needs as threatening and problematic. On the other hand, if your childhood needs were responded to with anger, irritation, neglect, rejection; if your early experience taught you that needs are *bad* and trigger negative feelings in those you rely on, and therefore lead to the loss of safety and love, you will most likely build a suspicious and critical relationship with your internal world.

In this chapter, I present different family environments that may be similar to yours. I touch on these lightly, really, to invite you into your own deeper investigation. Read these scenarios slowly, in increments, not all at once. Notice what each style of caretaking evokes in you. Where do you recognize yourself and your family?

Consider how *your* home environment shaped the way you relate to others in trying to get your needs met. Consider the ways that your caretakers responded to your needs and how that shaped the ways you respond to your needs. Ask yourself (kindly), *Am I still operating from the same assumptions and fears that made sense as a child? Am I still trying to protect myself from the dangers of my childhood home?*

Before moving on, acknowledge the difficulty you navigated and endured. And furthermore, the creative and maybe even ingenious ways you tried to take care of yourself—without the resources and awareness you needed to do so.

Out in the Cold

When you grow up in an environment in which your emotional needs are neglected, when what you receive from your caregivers is not a good fit for your particular emotional wiring, or when empathy is scarce, you learn to relate to your own feelings in a similar fashion—to shut down and disconnect from them. To go numb. You stop listening to and caring about your own experience. The assumption is that no one is there for you and nothing can be done to help you.

Patty remembers her childhood home as cold, emotionally and physically. The house she grew up in was big, but the space felt like it was filled with emptiness and a few people who barely knew each other. An only child, she was sensitive, a bit sad, and wired to feel things deeply. "It felt like the stork had dropped me in the wrong home; I belonged in a warm rainforest, but here I was growing up in an emotional tundra." Food was always on the table and her clothes were always clean and ironed; her father was a good provider on a practical level, but there wasn't anywhere or anyone to go to for connection or support, and certainly not anything as indulgent as empathy. As she poignantly described, "It was a home without a hug."

In the rare instances when she shared things like *not* getting invited to a friend's birthday party or finding out the popular girls were making fun of her, she described her mother's response as "painfully awkward... as if she had absolutely no idea what to say to me, and even less of an idea (if that's possible) of how to comfort me." Patty's mother would usually manage an icy pat on the back or a *you'll make other friends* kind of response. But nothing her mother offered brought real comfort or relief; nothing made Patty feel better, or loved for that matter. As a result, Patty felt fundamentally alone. She felt like a tolerated boarder floating around in her parents' home.

And indeed, what grows from such an environment is a deep belief that you are alone in the world, on your own when it comes to getting your needs met and in every other way. You become convinced that you're the only one you can rely on to take care of you. You may still believe that others want what's best for you, but in your gut, you don't believe that anyone can actually *help* you.

And so, you tuck away your feelings, share nothing that makes you feel vulnerable or causes you to reexperience your aloneness. On the inside, you become an emotional island. Sadly, you continue living your early experience, your early deprivation, long after you've moved out of your childhood home.

Too Much to Bear

Alternatively, if your caretakers were consistently overwhelmed by your needs, shaken by them, if they couldn't remain calm and emotionally intact in the face of your emotional needs, different defenses are born. You evolve into a woman for whom emotional needs are not just unwelcome, but also dangerous and potentially destructive.

Stephanie's mother was anxious, unstable, and emotionally fragile: "When I needed help or felt bad, my mother would become overwhelmed by my feelings and literally collapse into tears." When it came to helping Stephanie manage her experience, her mother was useless. Stephanie not only didn't receive the comfort and guidance she needed as a child, but her mother's emotional distress, frightening and destabilizing as it was, became another source of stress for Stephanie, another problem to manage on top of whatever she was already dealing with.

At the same time, Stephanie felt guilty for her needs. "I didn't want to make my mother cry, to burden her with my issues." Expressing needs actually made things worse, not better. And not just for herself, but seemingly for everyone involved.

Furthermore, when Stephanie approached her father with anything she couldn't solve or fix on her own, his first response was, *"Don't tell your mother."* "My father didn't want to have to deal with my mother's distress, to have to pick up the pieces after she heard about *my issues.*" Problems and emotional needs, Stephanie came to understand, were dangerous affairs. Stephanie's needs disrupted not only her mother's well-being, but her father's as well. Her needs were harmful to the two people she needed most and most needed to be okay. Her needs were in conflict with each other—as is so often the case.

If you grew up like Stephanie, being vulnerable resulted in an emotional mess, which led to guilt and shame for having made that mess and caused pain in those you loved and needed. With this as a foundation, you probably learned to keep your needs bottled up and only present them when they were light and easy, or when you had them all figured out. You discovered that it was safer to share your needs once you were no longer in need, when you could present your problem tied up with a bow, as yet another example of something you'd experienced but now, thankfully, solved on your own.

This early experience teaches you that your needs will flood and consume those you rely on and love, which is a confusing message at any age. You learn that other people are unable to provide you with solid footing and support, to comfort and hold *you* in your state of vulnerability. Guidance and help, you understand quickly, are out of the question. And so, sadly, you come to see your own needs as overwhelming and unmanageable, capable of destroying anyone who stands in their wake. The conclusion, then, is that *you* are the only one who can handle your own needs.

If you were raised in this kind of emotional ecosystem, you may have become a master people pleaser, the sort of woman who is really good at making everyone happy. *Not okay*, as you would have learned, is not okay, and so you make sure it doesn't happen.

At the same time, you may have become highly efficient and independent, the kind of woman who always has it all together and always takes care of her own needs, or simply doesn't have any. People-pleasing and resourcefulness become your coping strategies and a way to prevent having to relive the suffering you experienced with your early caretakers. Caretaking becomes your way to be liked and accepted; it becomes a trait on which to base your self-esteem and identity.

And it works, to a point. But unfortunately, while it may keep you safe and even make you feel strong, the people-pleasing, *having it all together* strategy is ultimately unsatisfying. Plus, like these other compensatory behaviors, it continues the pattern of your childhood, whereby your own needs are never sufficiently met.

"What Now?!"

Let's consider another kind of home environment now, one that's unfortunately quite common: the blaming environment. Did your needs consistently trigger irritation and anger in your caretakers, even the withdrawal of love? Were your needs an irritant and a bother to your caretakers? And worse, did your needs make *you* an irritant and a bother—or even a target?

When Kara was not okay, when she needed any kind of help or comfort, her father would angrily bark, "What now?" Her needs triggered wrath; she was scolded and often punished for being upset. Her caretakers experienced her needs not only as *a pain in the ass,* but also as something that she was deliberately doing *to them.* "My needs were my fault, for upsetting *their* world." But because she was young and had no other frame of reference, no experience with which to compare it; because her parents' response was understood (as it is for children) as just how life was, and what love looked like, she did what we all do: corrected *her* behavior. When what's normal in a family is not normal, the children figure out how to be, well...not normal.

If you grew up this way, you likely associate your needs with guilt and fear, and also shame: there is something wrong with you when you have needs; needs make the people you care about mad at you. Put simply, needs mean you'll be rejected. And so, for relationships to feel secure, and to meet your need to be loved, you learn to bury your needs—to bury *you*—which then causes you to be emotionally shut down and unfulfilled. Denying your needs ultimately becomes unsustainable, as you can't feel loved if you don't feel seen or known and if your needs are not welcome.

Not Your Needs Too

The conviction that your needs are an irritant is not unique to angry households. With busy and preoccupied parents, you may form a similarly fearful and unfriendly relationship with your own needs.

Nina's memory of her childhood home was that it was always in a state of chaos and she was always in the way. As she described, no one had the bandwidth for anything as insignificant as the feelings or needs of a child, a child who had no job and no real stressors, as they saw it. The adults were so busy and stressed out making ends meet and putting out fires, it would have been ridiculous and indulgent—greedy, in fact— for her to ask more from them. Nina would have been yet another problem for her parents to deal with, and there were already too many problems. There was no room for her emotional needs; to need anything would have meant asking for time and attention her caretakers didn't have to give.

With caretakers so overwhelmed, overburdened, and self-involved, Nina felt guilty even though she didn't know what she was guilty for. "I felt guilty—just for existing." The takeaway was that it was more considerate (and wiser) to keep her needs to herself so as not to add more problems to her parents' already problem-filled lives. Nina (like all of us) wanted to be loved and seen as good—*not* a problem. In her family, and in so many families, being loved meant taking care of her caretakers—by leaving them alone and not asking for the care she really needed.

When you grow up with overwhelmed and preoccupied caretakers, you build a sense of worth and an identity based on your ability to take care of yourself. Your self-esteem gets linked with your ability to *not* need and *not* be a problem. Ultimately, to be invisible except for what makes other people happy. Often, you are praised and respected precisely for this ability to be *need-less* and never ask for help. "She's so good...she never needs a thing; she can do it all by herself. She makes it so easy for us!" You are loved, or so it feels, precisely for your capacity to *not* need in an environment in which you intuitively know there's no room to need.

With such a history, it can take a long time to trust that your worth is not based on your ability to be completely self-sufficient—to exist without any needs. It takes a lot of healing to believe that you could ever be loved in such a way that your needs would *not* be experienced as a problem.

Your Needs, Your Fault

Sadly, blame takes many forms in families—none of them loving or helpful. You may have experienced a home in which your needs were used against you, as an opportunity to criticize you and point out your faults.

For Adriana, admitting that she wasn't okay led to an immediate assessment of her flaws. The message from her parents was that whatever problems, feelings, or needs she had, *she* was the cause of them. *She* was too sensitive, too needy, got hurt too easily, had a broken pain threshold, expected too much from people, couldn't just accept people the way they were, wanted too much…and the list went on. Regardless of the problem, the solution was always the same: Adriana needed to change—to fix who she was.

Not surprisingly, when Adriana experienced strong emotions, she immediately felt shame. Her needs were evidence of her inadequacy and everything else that was wrong and unlovable about her. Expressing needs left her with a long list of faults to correct and a heavy dose of self-loathing and shame. And certainly no help or support. Consequently, she learned to shut down her emotional needs before they had a chance to fully form. Over time, she became a woman who didn't have to feel wrong and unlovable, but also didn't get to feel much of anything.

When you grow up in this kind of home, you often become an adult with a highly accommodating and sometimes falsely positive persona. Simultaneously, you become someone who's afraid to express your real feelings. You learn to take care of your own needs or pretend they don't exist…to keep your real feelings to yourself. Ultimately, you become someone who's always *okay*, because if you're not, there's only one person to blame—you.

"What About Me?"

In yet another kind of home, the expression of needs unleashes a hornet's nest of a parent's own emotional baggage.

Serena's memory of needing, or just not being okay, was that it led to a self-hating and regretful rant from her mother. How terrible a parent her mother had been, how deficient a human being, and how badly she had failed Serena (which was the reason Serena was not okay). Serena's needs were responded to through the lens of what they suggested about her mother, which was either a condemnation of her parenting or her character. Serena's upset triggered her mother's self-loathing and remorse, which naturally made Serena feel guilty and responsible for her mother's suffering.

It also triggered anger in Serena; just as her mother was lamenting having failed her in the past, she was actively failing her and refusing to parent her in the present moment. As Serena described, "It got to where I wouldn't share anything difficult, any emotional needs, because I just couldn't listen to how much she hated herself and how my experience was all because of her and how she'd failed. My feelings were always all about *her*…never about me. So, it's not like I was going to *get* anything by sharing."

When you grow up in a home in which your feelings and needs are experienced as narcissistic injuries to your caretakers, as all *about* your caretakers—how your needs make *them* feel—you learn, simply, to stop sharing. It's not worth making your parent feel bad or being flooded with their guilt and self-loathing. It's also not worth having your experience hijacked by your parent and realizing, again, how un-parented you really are. You've learned that your experience can never just be about *you*; it's always about the other in one way or another. Doing away with your needs, or at least keeping them to yourself, then becomes the path of least suffering.

The Perils of Virtue: Be Strong or Be Weak— You Choose

All families have characteristics and virtues that they respect and ideal-ize, even if they're never spoken about. You probably could tell me, without having to think much, what qualities made a person admirable and good in the eyes of your caretakers. As it turns out, this system of values, and what your family respected, also ends up playing an impor-tant role in the relationship you build with your own needs and how you allow or don't allow your needs to be known—by others and yourself.

Willow was reared in a family with a classic Protestant work ethic. Strong and resourceful were the ultimate compliments that could be bestowed on a person. Those considered self-sufficient, diligent, and independent, who asked for and needed nothing, were the ones most admired and adored by her caretakers. The ability to meet challenges head-on without a whimper, and without inconveniencing or putting anyone else out, was considered a virtue of the highest order. The better you were at figuring it out on your own, the better *you* were considered to be.

One of Willow's favorite memories was of the day when her mother offhandedly referred to her as a *toughie*. It was the ultimate compliment, and the moment Willow knew she was not just respected, but actually loved; she'd won a real place in her mother's heart. It was also the moment that she had permission to view herself in this positive light.

With this as her early template, the adult Willow, not surprisingly, was a self-sufficient and resilient woman. Exposing emotional needs was not an option for her. Emotional needs were an admission that she was weak and couldn't make it on her own, which destroyed any possibility of being seen as strong and independent, which she desperately wanted to be. Strength and needs were mutually exclusive.

Consequently, Willow learned to deny her needs; she handled them on her own without *whining about it* or expecting anyone to help. In her words, "My needs are my responsibility." Most important for Willow was that she stay true to the *toughie* her mother loved, and to the kind of person that her mother *could* love.

Being emotionally strong is a quality that many families value and respect. To be strong is to be worthy and admirable; the ability to withstand hardship without complaint is considered a noble trait in our culture. But being strong, if you're not careful, can also be conflated with not having needs—as in, you're weak when you have needs and strong when you don't. You then accept these familial values as fundamental truths, and consequently, discard and discount your needs so they won't reflect poorly on your image and identity.

Selfless as a Badge of Honor

Like many girls, Betsy's model for how to be a virtuous woman came from watching her mother, which meant watching her mother take care of the family. Betsy's experience of her mother was that she was created to take care of others: "Serving was the purpose of her existence."

But at the same time, her mother didn't appear to be a fully formed person in her own right—someone with her own wants and needs. Betsy had no idea who her mother really was. As she put it, "My mother was someone who lived to make sure everyone else got what *they* needed. In fact, for a long time, my sisters and I assumed that she dematerialized when we weren't there."

Simultaneously, Betsy's mother modeled a way of being in a relationship that was absent of an independent self. For years, her mother stood by as Betsy's father disappeared into an addiction to pain medications. Betsy's parents lived together in a state of denial and passivity, with no one taking responsibility for his or her own life. To assume responsibility for one's own needs in this family dynamic would have been to establish one's self as separate and autonomous, which would have been disloyal and an abandonment of the merger that defined their partnership. The relationship was set up to remain as one indivisible unit, with no possibility for two separate selves.

When you grow up with this kind of self-less mother or other female figure as a model, you learn to view your own needs as a betrayal of the larger family unit and those you love. You come to believe that you don't have the right to your own needs. Who are *you* to get to take care of your own needs…what makes *you* so special? Would that really be fair, when your mother devoted her entire life to and gave up everything for you? Long after you leave your childhood home, you may still believe that you're supposed to dedicate your life to the service of others; you may still feel guilty for attending to your own needs.

But Am I Worth It, Really?

Perhaps the most important truth you can learn in your childhood home is that you are fundamentally deserving of love, and that your worth is not because of anything you do, accomplish, or offer, and not something you have to earn or prove; your value is inherent to who you are—inarguable and irrevocable, simply because you *are*. Nurturing this knowing in a child is in fact the most important aspect of caretaking. But sadly, in my experience, few of us receive this kind of love; few of us genuinely believe that we are worthy—fundamentally worthy. To emerge from childhood with a trust in your unconditional and inarguable value—not for what you do, but for who you are—is the exception, not the rule.

When I met Gina, I was taken by what a lovely and lovable woman she was. Ironically, one of the first things she said was this: "Any time I ask a friend for something, even if it's just to spend time with me, to listen, I feel like I have to bring them muffins—to at least offer them *something*, I guess, to be worthy of their time." So many of us feel, like

Gina, that we have to offer more than just ourselves, *do* something extra that's *for* the other person. *We* are not enough on our own, and so we have to make sure there's something *in it* for them.

When you're raised in an environment that fails to offer you this basic sense of worthiness, this trust in your inherent value; when you emerge from childhood feeling not good enough, or just plain not enough, you are naturally inclined to believe that your needs are also unworthy and undeserving. Your needs are not important because *you* are not important. *Why would anyone care about what I want and need? Why would I care?* You can easily recognize that other people's needs are important and deserving of attention and care, but *your* needs? *That* is hard to believe.

Understand Your Past, Choose Your Present

The way your needs were attended to as a child and the way you experienced your needs through the lens of your caretakers set the tone for how you respond to your own needs as an adult. I hope by now that's clear. However, if you're not conscious of your own history, your early experiences can lock you into a way of being that's counterproductive and unhealthy. As you unpack your emotional exhaustion, you cannot ignore your early environment; it's where your beliefs about needs were born and grew and where you learned to twist your needs into distorted shapes so as to try and get them met. It's where, ultimately, we determined what we need to do to belong—and survive.

In presenting these archetypal environments, I'm inviting you to get curious about your own early experience and coping strategies around needs. While the prompts below may all sound similar, they will jostle loose different truths if taken in slowly and one at a time. Contemplate these questions, and always, always, always be curious and kind with whatever comes in response.

In your childhood home...

How were your needs and feelings responded to?

What did it feel like to ask your caretakers for help or comfort?

What did your needs and feelings elicit in your caregivers? Were there consequences for asking for what you needed or being honest about your feelings? If so, what were they, and how did you respond?

What were the spoken and unspoken beliefs about needs and about the people who had expressed them?

How do you think your early experience with caretakers affects the way you try and get your needs met now?

How does it affect the way you relate to your own needs?

The purpose of this is to get to know the soil in which your needs originally grew, or got stamped out or starved. To become aware of the ways in which ignoring, stuffing down, or judging your needs may have kept you safe at another time (and therefore been a wise adaptation).

Know this: You didn't come into this world afraid, angry, or distrustful of yourself; you weren't born into an unfriendly relationship with your own needs. You were born with a self-protective and self-caring nature; you entered this life on your own side. And yet, you may have learned to replace your natural instincts with an unnatural and unhealthy way of being with yourself—paradoxically, to stay safe and thereby take care of yourself. But here's the good news: the inherent self-protector in you, the healthy one you were born *with*, is still there in you, waiting to be invited back in.

Taught to Fear

There's a reason we view our needs as dangerous, and it's not because they *are* dangerous or because it's enjoyable or easy to relate to them as such. It's neither enjoyable nor easy to reject our own experience. We reject our needs because our lived experience has taught us that needs are a threat to being loved, that when our needs enter our most important relationships, they create conflict and difficulty. We learn that a cautious and controlling relationship with our needs keeps us safe in the ecosystem in which we're trying to survive. We determine that it's smoother and more productive to take care of others than it is to take care of ourselves. It becomes our habit and way of being in the world.

But most of all, we learn that our deepest need, the need to belong, is endangered by our other needs. And so, we choose the path that will bring us what matters most, what we need the most—to stay safe and be loved. This need-less path then becomes the paradigm by which we live.

But awareness is the kryptonite to our habitual patterning, the light we shine into ourselves so that we can see those behaviors we keep acting out because we imagine that they still protect us. Once you become aware of your early conditioning, how your needs were responded to by your caretakers—what your family valued and how these factors shaped your behaviors and beliefs; once you can see the ways you learned to manage yourself so as to try and get your needs met, then you're on your way to emotional freedom. You're in the process of creating a different relationship with yourself.

Armed with greater clarity and awareness, you can decide whether it's necessary to keep relating to your environment through the same lens and with the same coping strategies that made sense as a child. You can consider whether you have different resources and greater wisdom now, and therefore can take care of yourself in ways you couldn't when you were younger. With awareness, you can see the fears and resulting behaviors that stemmed from your experience with your family of origin. You can also recognize how those behaviors may no longer be needed, useful, or healthy for you, and no longer how you *want* to behave.

When you see a belief and understand its origin, you no longer have to keep unconsciously acting it out. Once again, with awareness comes freedom.

Going Beyond the Matrix

Thus far, we've been considering societal messaging and family conditioning, the pervasive narratives and early experiences that weave together into an elaborate web of conscious and unconscious beliefs about needs. This complex and intricate matrix of perceived truths we imagine to be reality then shapes how we respond to ourselves and our own experience. Such external forces, which become internal forces, ultimately determine what we think we're allowed to feel and express—or maybe more blatantly, *not* allowed to feel or express. These forces help us formulate not only the strategies we live *by*, but also the emotional cage we live *in*.

From here, we'll venture deeper into the shadowed corners of the mind where your core beliefs are nesting; we'll set out to unearth the truths you assume about your needs, without even knowing you're assuming them. The core beliefs that, ultimately, are controlling your life.

4

CORE BELIEFS

The strange reality is that we're all, every single one of us, walking around carrying a backpack full of ideas and beliefs about the way the world works and what's True. The contents of our backpacks are all different, based on what we've lived, but strangely, we think that they're the same. Until we unpack our own baggage, however, and see the beliefs we're believing and the reality we're imagining, we remain stuck in the same narratives, relating to the world and ourselves in the same way we always have—whether it *works* for us or not. We will continue living an unconscious and unintentional life, driven by our unformulated and shadowed beliefs—until, that is, we can bring our beliefs into the light, understand their origin, and question their veracity. Thankfully, most of us reach a point where it simply hurts too much to keep operating from the same beliefs.

Perhaps you're in enough pain now to change things…if so, that's a good thing (even though it doesn't feel good). With enough exhaustion and dissatisfaction, you will start wondering whether you still want to believe your operating truths and if they were ever actually true. And so, the question begs: What are the core beliefs that make caring about yourself feel so dangerous, shameful, and counterintuitive?

Getting to the Core of Core Beliefs

Our core beliefs are hard to see; these deep-seated ideas about the way the world works and what's possible for us are so interwoven into our psyche as to render them nearly imperceptible. They are the truths we never question because they feel like *what is*...the Truth. Core beliefs don't feel like beliefs; they don't feel separate from us. They feel like who we are. Our core beliefs reside and hide inside the very lens through which we perceive the world. They are the fabric out of which our narratives—the meanings we make and the stories we tell ourselves—are woven. Ultimately, they run the show that is our life. And yet, remarkably, we don't see them, these powerful forces—until we go looking for them and turn the lens on our own lens. With awareness, we can recognize our core beliefs as just ideas we've been conditioned to believe, stories we've built out of self-selected experiences—but not what's true, and certainly not who we are.

In this chapter, I discuss some of the common beliefs that women hold. You may be carrying a few of them around too, in varying degrees. Your work is to recognize these core beliefs in you, to separate them from who you are, and from the Truth. You bring them to light so that you can decide what you want to do with them, rather than their deciding what they want to do with *you*. The goal, ultimately, is to become aware of these beliefs you are acting from and acting out. To open that backpack and see what's been in there all along—and then, miraculously, drop it.

Belief: I Am Choosing My Needs

Sarah sat in the back seat with her four-year-old son. Her mother-in-law was at the wheel. It had been a fun, albeit exhausting, day at the amusement park. Eight hours of spinning airplane rides, nausea, hot dogs, meltdowns, cotton candy, and long, shadeless lines in the blazing sun.

Not to mention endless trips to the too-small-for-two portable toilet. Sarah was exhausted and more than a little parented-out.

Gazing out the window, Sarah noticed that they would soon be passing her favorite vineyard. She started imagining the bright green and orange Adirondack chairs on the vineyard's lush lawn. She pictured herself, glass of wine in hand, relaxing into the sounds of the bluegrass band that would just be starting their happy hour set. It was where every cell in her body wanted to be.

Suddenly, she was overtaken with an intense wanting; it felt like a snake uncoiling inside her spine. She hungered for an experience, a moment that was *for* her—not her as a mother, daughter-in-law, wife, nor any of the countless other roles she played for the people in her life. She needed a moment of enjoyment, whose value was not derived from what it would offer someone else (*this makes me happy because it makes my son happy*), or what it would say about her (*this makes me a good mother*), or any other means to any other end. Sarah was craving, as she succinctly put it, "Something I actually *want* to do."

Sarah's mother-in-law then announced that they would be stopping off at the grocery store to pick up chicken nuggets since they had finished them the night before. She also reminded Sarah that she should start getting her son's dinner ready as soon as they were home as it was already late.

With the vineyard disappearing in the minivan's taillights, a strong energy began rising up in Sarah's chest, as if that same snake were trying to climb into her throat. She felt resentful, of her son, her mother-in-law, her husband, and everyone who had created this system that kept her imprisoned in the back seat, behaving appropriately.

Within seconds, however, that snake had turned back around and bitten her—injecting its self-critical toxin into her system. The words that came were these: *Why are you choosing to be unhappy, to ruin this moment? Why can't you just focus on what you're getting rather than what you're not getting? Why can't you ever just be happy with what you have? Think of all the women who don't get to have any of this!*

But it didn't stop there; the venom kept coming. *It should be enough to spend this day with your child—to enjoy his enjoyment; why do you always need something for yourself? Your needs are proof that you're ungrateful and selfish—a bad mother.*

Sarah's core belief is that her needs are of her own making—chosen and fabricated—by her. And therefore, her needs can and should be changed. Like Sarah, you may hold yourself responsible for creating your negative feelings, thinking that you must be choosing to want what you shouldn't want. Or that it's your decision to be unhappy, to suffer. Your needs are thus evidence of your unworthiness, your impossible-to-please–ness. If you were less greedy, less negative, less resentful—a better person—then you would choose a different way to feel. You would want what you have. If you were different, you would be capable of experiencing life the way you *should* experience it. With the core belief that your feelings are something you're deciding to cook up, you then blame yourself for your own suffering.

Belief: My Needs Are the Cause of My Pain

Tess arrived home after an upsetting day; her boss had misinterpreted something she said, and the whole thing blew up into a situation that potentially threatened her upcoming promotion. She was upset and wanted to talk about it, so she poured herself a giant glass of wine and flopped onto the couch next to her husband. He listened to her vent for a minute or two then began showing his usual signs of boredom and irritation, "of having listened to my feelings long enough." As was his pattern, he reminded Tess that she knew how unreasonable her boss was. And then came the *shoulds*...she shouldn't be surprised or upset by her boss's nastiness, shouldn't let it get to her, and shouldn't expect anything else. She should be happy to just have a job. Boiled down, she shouldn't feel what she felt or need what she needed—from her boss (or her husband, for that matter).

When the conversation ended soon after, Tess now could add frustrated and hurt to the list of painful feelings she already felt. She was aching to be heard and not judged, to share not just the bullet points of the story, but what it felt like and what she needed now, none of which had been allowed in her allotted time before her husband's tolerance for her emotional needs expired. What Tess really needed was a place where *all* of her was welcome, where, in her words, she "didn't have to focus on not being too repetitive, too emotional, too boring, too needy, too demanding, or too anything else to be cared about." Nonetheless, in her state of loneliness, Tess did what she always did: she tucked her needs away, stuffed them down, and soldiered on. She went back to being a version of herself that maintained peace in the relationship, back to being *just fine*—with anything and everything.

Later that night, Tess sensed a heaviness in her chest; it felt like grief. She was emotionally exhausted, with the growing conviction that she would never receive what she really needed, from anyone. Her mind returned to the conversation with her husband. She felt heartbroken— for herself. But immediately, upon recognizing her own exhaustion and sensing her own grief, Tess turned against herself. Here's what she heard inside her head: *Why is my husband's perfectly reasonable wish to have a nice dinner at the end of his long day such a problem for me? Why do I demand that everyone be able to understand my experience so precisely? Why can't I just let this go?* And the real punch: *Why do I keep doing this to myself—and him?* Like so many women, Tess believed that her experience was something she was doing *to* herself; she was creating her needs and thus creating her pain.

These two related core beliefs—*I choose my feelings and therefore should be able to change them* and *My feelings (and needs) are why I suffer* (both so common among women)—come together to play an important role in your relationship with your own experience. Armed with the conviction that you are to blame for your feelings, it feels threatening and counterintuitive to acknowledge your experience with kindness. Why would you ever empathize with feelings that you're creating, which cause you to suffer? To do so would be to encourage and strengthen a part of yourself that's destructive. As you imagine it, you could choose a different experience than the one you're having; you could choose to be happy. Acknowledging and attending to your actual experience, therefore, would be a move in the wrong direction, like inviting an unwanted and dangerous intruder in for tea.

And so you reject your feelings and return to what is, for many women, a favorite question: *What's wrong with me that I feel this way and have these needs?* And around and around you go, with your needs still unmet and yourself still to blame.

Belief: I Shouldn't Need What I Need

When I first met Kelsey, she spent her weekends on hold, waiting for her partner to become available so they could do something together. When he wasn't free, she did "a whole lot of nothing." But she started to feel bored and uncomfortable with this situation, and ashamed by how little she knew about her own interests. As she said, "Sometimes I don't feel as if I have a self, as if I *am* someone, I mean of my own, not in relation to the person I'm dating."

I was curious about Kelsey, which allowed her to become more curious about herself. She got interested in finding out what she enjoyed, and what inspired her. Surprisingly, she realized that she loved yoga and felt strongly drawn to meditation. For the first time ever, Kelsey began to feel alive, engaged, and confident; she began to feel like someone who existed *on her own*. She discovered that a few minutes of meditation and yoga practice, followed by her own self-brewed blend of teas, set her up for a day of feeling present, grounded, and happy—a day of feeling like *herself.*

The relationship with her boyfriend did not survive her evolution, however. For her partner, the always-available Kelsey, the one without interests or needs, was preferable and more desirable than the defined and grounded version of her, the version who existed separate from him.

A few months later, a new boyfriend appeared, and Kelsey started spending weekends at his house. At the beginning of their courtship, she maintained a strong and consistent yoga, meditation, and tea practice. She knew that she needed to connect regularly with her body and herself and to pay attention to her own needs in order to be well. This knowing was indisputable…at the beginning of the relationship.

Within a few weeks, however, the aroma of an old belief system began wafting through our conversations. Kelsey had stopped talking about her self-care practices, which just weeks before she had called "nonnegotiable." Apparently it just wasn't practical to self-care at her boyfriend's house in the ways she needed to. To begin with, there wasn't any place to store her tea or unroll her yoga mat. But even if those issues could be solved, Kelsey worried her boyfriend would think she was "a woo-woo girl," if he knew all the things she needed "just to function." Her self-care practices, which had been so meaningful and helpful to her, were now reframed through (what she imagined to be) her boyfriend's lens. As a result, her needs had lost their value and subsequently went out the window. Her needs were only legitimate if he saw them as legitimate, and he didn't.

Soon, Kelsey had stopped doing what she needed to do for herself during the work week as well. Not surprisingly, she was feeling increasingly irritable, defensive, and anxious. Her sense of liking and trusting herself, knowing what she needed, was also slipping away.

"But I should be able to be okay and *be* myself without all my rituals," she said cynically. "Who needs a special tea just to feel okay? My boyfriend doesn't need a thousand rituals just to function. He gets up, showers, and goes to work, like a normal person." The problem, as she saw it, was not that she wasn't doing her practices, but the fact that she needed them in the first place.

This core belief tells her that she shouldn't need what she needs. She then refuses to acknowledge her needs because they're the wrong needs, and *she's* wrong for having them. Like Kelsey, you may claim that you will take care of yourself once you need what you *should* need, and once you become the person who feels the right way—what you *should* feel. But unfortunately, for most women, those right feelings never come. And consequently, the person you are now, with the feelings you actually have, is deprived of what she needs.

Belief: I'll Take Care of Myself When I Become Someone Who Deserves to Be Taken Care Of

Lisa hailed from Southern California, but had lived in Minnesota for nearly a decade, a place she described as "brutally cold, with a winter that's not technically a season since it lasts the entire year." Lisa was also an avid runner. Running was her greatest joy. She confessed that she needed to run just to feel like a human and have the patience to interact with other humans, and to feel any kind of peace with herself. But with the ground covered in snow and ice much of the year, coupled with the dark and frigid mornings, Lisa found that it was too hard to keep up her running regimen. Without the running, though, she felt lethargic and uninspired, depressed—and she had felt that way for years.

Knowing that Lisa had financial means, I asked her why she didn't join a gym so that she could run indoors during the coldest months. She told me flat-out that joining a gym wasn't an option because she should be able to run outside, should be the kind of person who can do what needs to be done, even if it's hard. As she viewed it, she shouldn't need to join a gym to be able to run. The person who was limited by the cold and unwilling to venture out in the frigid mornings was not someone whose needs she would consider. That person could remain lethargic, uninspired, and glum for all she cared. Years later, Lisa was still waiting to become the person who was disciplined enough to exercise outside, the person she should be, who would be deserving of her care and whose well-being she would then take seriously.

Lisa had tried desperately to become a woman who could drag herself out in the dark, icy mornings, but the problem was, she *wasn't* that woman and probably wasn't ever going to be her. Are you expecting yourself to become someone different, better, worthy—the someone you should be? Do you need this to happen before you'll grant yourself permission to take care of yourself? Consider how long you've been waiting, and how long you're going to keep waiting, to become someone else before you're willing to start caring about yourself. When will the woman you actually are be deserving of your care? When does your experience in this moment get to matter? The truth is, you can start relating to yourself as someone who matters—right now—in your fully unfinished and utterly imperfect form. What if, just as you are, you're already deserving of your own care…? You are.

Belief: Having Needs Means I Don't Appreciate What I Have

My friend Abby had just celebrated a birthday. For her special day, her husband and children treated her to a celebratory dinner out. As was the family tradition, the restaurant they chose was a surprise until they arrived at their destination. When she pulled off her blindfold that evening (part of the tradition), Abby discovered that she was standing in front of one of the most expensive and hard-to-get-a-reservation sushi restaurants in their city. It drew mostly businesspeople and other corporate expense accounts because of the outlandish prices. The hostess informed them that the family would be having dinner in their streatery, otherwise known as a table on the street, with automobile exhaust and noise as part of their extravagant experience.

For Abby, this restaurant, this expense, this noise, this experience—all of it was dreadful. Abby liked casual, quiet, un-sceney spots. She preferred simple dishes and generous portions over the micro-size, uber-fancy plates for which this chef was famous. Furthermore, she was fully aware that her husband's income did not accommodate prices like these, at least not without giving up other things that he needed, which would stress him out, and in the long run, come back to haunt her in other ways. The whole celebration felt like an exercise in inauthenticity and obligation—a performance. As her family studied her for evidence of delight to confirm that they had chosen well, Abby silently wrestled with the urge to sob. She knew that she was deeply loved, and at the same time, she had never felt so deeply alone.

Abby was faced with what felt like an impossible choice. She was grateful for the effort her family had put into making this night happen, filled with love and appreciation for her husband and daughters and their attempts to make her happy. Still, she didn't want any of this, not one single bit of it. What she wanted was an experience that she didn't have to pretend to want so that her family could feel good about themselves and not be disappointed by her disappointment. She wondered who her birthday was really for—her or them? As far back as she could remember, her birthday (and every other day, it seemed) had been about making sure that everyone felt good about themselves and proud of their efforts. The whole dance and ritual of self-abandonment was exhausting.

Abby stayed quiet and ate her $300 plate of raw fish, appropriately oohing and aahing at its deliciousness...afraid that if she spoke up and shared her real truth, her family would feel rejected and unappreciated, and that she would spoil their evening and be seen as the "Debbie Downer who ruins everything nice." Her birthday dinner left her feeling trapped and sad, unable and unwilling to be authentic with those she loved the most and who she most wanted to truly *know* her. Even though it was supposedly *her* day, Abby felt compelled to give her family the experience they needed rather than giving herself the experience she needed.

Many of us, like Abby, maybe like you too, operate from the core belief that needing something other than what's being offered means that we can't—also—feel appreciation and gratitude for what's offered. You may be convinced that you cannot want something else and also appreciate what you have. When faced with two seemingly contradictory truths, you insert a *but* between the two truths. *I am deeply grateful for your efforts—but—I need something else. I love you—but—I don't love this.* The word *but*, used in this way, is an eraser word; it effectively wipes out everything that came before it—in this case, acknowledgment of their kindness, appreciation, and gratitude. And yet, contradictory truths can coexist; two seemingly contrasting truths can be separated by an *and*. "I am deeply grateful for your efforts—*and*—I have other needs."

Belief: If I Acknowledge My Needs, I'll Fall Apart

Gina had always been a doer—competent, resilient, and resourceful. She had three young kids, a good marriage, close friends, and a career she enjoyed. She took great care of everyone in her life, and for all intents and purposes her life was *working*. Still, like many women, she felt weary and wiped out. Choking back tears, she confessed that she *also* wanted to be taken care of: "I'm embarrassed to admit it, but sometimes I want to receive the kind of care that I provide, the kind that happens without anyone having to ask for it or explain what they need; it just happens because I'm paying close attention to them. I want to be taken care of without asking too."

When I asked Gina what got in the way of receiving this kind of care, she surprised me with her answer. She said that she couldn't possibly *risk* letting herself be taken care of because if she did, she would completely fall apart. Allowing herself to feel how much she wanted and needed caretaking would lead to her collapse; her needs would be a bottomless pit, unending, which would mean, most importantly, that she wouldn't be able to fulfill her numerous responsibilities to other people. Gina was clear: getting everything done that she needed to get done, taking care of everyone that she needed to take care of, without question required that she ignore her own needs—most of all, her need to be taken care of.

Like Gina, you may believe that letting yourself be taken care of would render you useless—that either you can be taken care of or you can take care of others, but not both. And yet, this is a false belief. In fact, when you deny yourself the opportunity to be taken care of and keep silent on your need for care, you end up rejecting exactly the experience that would replenish and restore you. In a misguided effort to fulfill your responsibilities to others, you ignore your responsibility to yourself. As a result, your exhaustion and loneliness intensify. In reality (as opposed to our conditioned belief system), taking care of others becomes easier and more satisfying when you admit and acknowledge your own humanness and start showing up as a real person—with real needs and even, dare I say it, limitations. The fact is, a well-taken-care-of *you* makes for a less depleted, less resentful, and more genuine caretaker. Receiving and giving can form a most beautiful handshake, if you will let them.

Belief: I Don't Deserve Good Things

"Paying attention to my own needs? That would imply that I deserve, well...anything." Hallie went on, "It would mean that I'm worthy of being cared about and have a right to what I want. Do I really deserve it? I'm not so sure." Hallie's core belief of *I don't deserve anything good* is the most prevalent and damaging of all our core beliefs and one that we hold onto with the most ferocious tenacity.

The assumption that you matter and are deserving of care may not be one you entirely agree with or agree with at all. In fact, the complete opposite may be true for you. *What have I done to earn my so-called worthiness?* may be the question that makes the most sense to you, as it is for so many women. The idea that you could care about yourself just because you matter, and not because of what you give or provide, is likely a challenging premise to accept.

Cleverly, however, we've come up with a backdoor solution to the problem of our unworthiness so as to be able to get at least a little bit of what we need. We brilliantly created the narrative that in order to take care of other people's needs, we must first take care of our own; we can't fill other people's buckets unless we fill our own bucket first. This then makes it our responsibility to take care of ourselves—so that we can be of service to others, which gives us a rationalization for taking care of ourselves that's acceptable, even if we still feel guilty about it.

This rationale gives you permission to pay attention to your own needs under the guise that it's not really about you (because nothing should be just about *you*). You should take care of yourself because it makes you a better caretaker.

While this *fill your own bucket* narrative is useful and true, it's not the same thing as taking care of yourself because you are inherently worthy, because you *deserve* to be taken care of—just because.

Belief: Having to Self-Care Means I'm Doing Something Wrong

Yet another core belief women struggle with is that taking care of our own needs is not something we should *have* to do for ourselves.

"Everyone's supposed to have someone to take care of them." "We're not supposed to do this for ourselves, it's not natural." "It feels like a punishment." "I'm tired of always having to take care of my own needs, I shouldn't have to, it's not fair." I hear these statements daily. We are convinced that attending to our own needs is proof that we're not getting the love we deserve, the love we imagine everyone else is getting, and that we're *supposed* to get. Certainly, in all the fairy tales, someone else takes care of the woman.

Deep down, you may believe that you shouldn't *have* to take care of yourself and that there's something wrong with you if you do. And furthermore, that you can't possibly get what you need from *just* yourself, that your own care is a paltry substitute for someone else's, the booby prize in what is most certainly a failed life. When you believe this, you turn your back on your own needs and refuse responsibility for your own care, stamping your figurative feet and demanding that someone else should be doing the job for you. To be responsible for yourself would be to accept defeat and render yourself a loser in the game of love. But the result is that you must live without your own attention, and consequently, *without* what you need.

Belief: It's Unfair for Me to Get My Needs Met When So Many Others Can't

One of the unexpected obstacles to getting our needs met, oddly, has to do with the issue of fairness. Women often ask me why it's okay for them to get their needs met when so many other people don't have that possibility, or luxury.

Wendy, after working for twenty years, decided to take a six-month sabbatical. She'd earned that time off and desperately needed it. But sadly, she spent the entire six months feeling guilty about her choice to take care of herself. Beating herself up for the privilege that she'd created. Wendy's core belief was that giving herself what she needed was unfair to those who couldn't get what *they* needed.

Like so many women, you may be conditioned to believe that you should never get more than someone else, and certainly never get something that someone else *can't* get. Reality should be fair, particularly when you're the one getting more than what you see as your fair share. This core belief causes you to reject an inarguable truth, namely, that life isn't fair and has never been fair—for anyone.

Some people are born with great intelligence, physical beauty, athletic prowess, and creative imagination. Some are born into wealth, supportive families, and opportunity. Others start with none of these gifts and arrive into social and emotional wastelands, or worse. Furthermore, our ability to respond to opportunities and challenges, to overcome obstacles and alchemize our gifts also varies widely. One person can make lemonade out of lemons while another can only drown in acidity. Our capacity for resilience, willingness to work hard, ability to make good choices, and attraction to the positive...it's all doled out in unfair and inequitable portions. Our opportunities as women are different just on account of being women. The fact is, we make our opportunities as best we can with what we're given and what we create.

Despite this undeniable truth, you may still believe that you shouldn't get to experience anything good that someone else doesn't get to experience. You may feel guilty and self-indulgent for allowing yourself to enjoy opportunities that others cannot enjoy, regardless of whether you earned those opportunities. Taking care of yourself in a system in which doing so is easier for some than others may feel like it's contributing to an unfairness that you don't deserve to benefit from. The inequities in life, the reality in reality—even *this* you're responsible and to blame for. As a result, you deny yourself possibilities, abandon your own self-care, all in a misguided attempt to assuage your guilt and make sure that you're not getting more than anyone else.

Belief: If I Take My Share, Someone Else Won't Get Theirs

A close cousin to this last belief is the conviction that if we receive what we want, accept our share of good things in life, then someone else will actually lose their share. In this frame, our getting is not just unfair, but also greedy and aggressive. Positive experiences are seen as finite resources, like that cookie we gave to our brother when we were five (and were so celebrated for doing). Accepting the goodies and creating what we want renders us guilty, yet again, as our win is someone else's loss. Essentially, we're taking more than our share. Ignoring our own wants and needs then, *doing without*, curiously, is seen as a backhanded service to those who are less fortunate or capable.

And yet, there is no zero-sum universe; we've made it up. The idea that ignoring our needs somehow balances out the unfairness of reality is another way for women to feel guilty and assume responsibility for what we're not responsible for and positively can't correct. Pretending that your needs don't matter will do nothing to even out the imbalances inherent in reality, nor give anyone else what they need. Imbalances will continue to exist whether you choose to take care of yourself or not. No one benefits from your denying yourself what you want and need. But one person definitely ends up losing, and that's you.

Belief: If My Needs Can't Be Met, I'm Better Off Not Knowing About Them

In the course of creating this book, I interviewed a multitude of women on the topic of needs. Throughout the process, I was continually asked the same question: *What's the point of becoming aware of my needs if I know those needs won't be met?* As one friend put it, "So, you want me to become more aware of what I'm never going to get? No thanks!"

The frequency and ferocity of this sentiment alerted me to another common belief we women hold. It goes like this: the only reason to pay attention to our own needs is if we know we're going to get them filled. If we might not get our needs met, or met in the ways we want them met, then we're better off *not* knowing they exist. Awareness will just make us feel worse—more deprived and even more depleted.

But in fact, awareness is the antidote to deprivation and the key to your freedom. To start with, once you can see the core beliefs from which you've been operating, the assumptions you've been holding as truths, and the ways you've been accommodating, solidifying, and reasserting such assumed truths, then you can start determining whether those beliefs are really true, if you still believe them, and if you *want* to keep believing and, most importantly, acting from such beliefs. At the same time, you can start, maybe for the first time, honoring and taking care of the needs that your core beliefs have convinced you are undeserving, unwanted, and unwise. With awareness, you are free to live and take care of yourself with a new level of conscious intention.

For anything in your life to change, you need one thing more than any other: awareness. You cannot create a new path until you can see the path you've been following and understand how you got to where you are.

So far, we've examined the judgments and labels that threaten women who express needs. We've looked at family dynamics that shape our fears and expectations around getting our needs met. And we've investigated internal core beliefs that determine the way we interact with our world. In short, we've been unpacking the mighty conditioning responsible for our conflicted, distrustful, and unfriendly attitude toward our own needs—and ultimately, toward ourselves.

For this problem, our society has invented a solution; we have a prescription for our current condition. We call it *self-care*, and it's where we'll venture next.

5

THE SELF-CARE "SOLUTION"

When Jenny showed up in my office, the only thing she knew for sure was that she was depleted and in desperate need of some sort of relief and replenishment. She had no idea how to get what she really needed to feel better, or *what* she needed for that matter. Soon after sharing this truth, however, her voice changed—noticeably. In a sharper and less kind tone, ironically, she announced that she planned to start taking better care of and being "kinder" to herself. As she put it, she needed to get better where her own needs were concerned.

In that first meeting I also learned that, as a teenager, Jenny had been diagnosed with a rare genetic condition that caused terrible stomach pain and a host of other debilitating symptoms. Her parents were dismissive of her condition and convinced, despite what the doctors explained, that her pain was *all in her head*. Her mother frequently told her not to make such a big deal of her stomachaches and accused her of needing attention and being dramatic. The result was that Jenny had spent her life trying hard not to need anything, and most certainly, not to need attention.

Now married, Jenny had not surprisingly chosen a man who vacillated between dismissing her pain, as her parents had, and blaming her for it. When she hurt, her husband told her to "just focus on something else," and continually reminded her of all the things she was doing wrong that created her pain. The message she received, once again, was that she was to blame for her suffering.

At the age of thirty-nine, Jenny had yet to encounter real comfort or care. Everywhere she'd tried to bring up her emotional needs, those needs had been rejected and judged as either illegitimate or her fault. When I met her, Jenny felt broken and undeserving of care. As far as she was concerned, her own suffering was unlovable, and worse, it made *her* unlovable. Her need for empathy and comfort, which had never been properly met, had long been shamed out of the room, and she was now the one doing the fiercest shaming.

At a loss for how to feel better, Jenny turned to self-care, hoping that *it* would take care of her. And indeed, she discovered a whole host of things she could do to feel better. Soon she was signed up for a spa retreat, a series of sound baths, and a color makeover for her wardrobe. She was going to learn to treat herself as if she mattered.

Three months later, having completed her first round of self-care treatments and programs, and now decked out in a new wardrobe of pastel tones and plush fabrics, Jenny reported feeling more limber, more aware of her body, calmer, and better dressed. She was five pounds lighter and carrying herself with more confidence...positive changes for sure.

And yet, while lighter and calmer, Jenny still felt lonely and guilty for her pain. A large part of her experience remained disallowed and abandoned. She still ached for an emotionally safe place where she could be honest and receive empathy instead of judgment. She still felt ashamed of her needs and angry at herself for being so needy and broken.

The self-care Jenny offered herself didn't take care of her at a deep level because it wasn't connected to who she was or what she really needed. Her self-care didn't *grow* from her; it wasn't informed by her real longings or experience. Everything she'd added to her life was good for her, but none of it touched the rejected and abandoned emotional needs at the core of her depletion. And it didn't heal her relationship with herself. Like many women, the care she offered herself was of the one-size-fits-all, outside-in variety, the generic prescription for the problem of not being okay. After months of diligently taking care of herself on the self-care industry's plan, Jenny still felt emotionally exhausted, only now the exhaustion came in a more limber and pastel package.

Since there are no clear statistics for what I'm calling emotional exhaustion, which includes so many different symptoms, let's investigate what's going on with women today under the umbrella term of *stress*. In a recent "Stress in America" report, 23 percent of women said that their stress levels are at an 8, 9, or 10 level, with 10 being a "great deal of stress."[1] All of this matches my research as well.

But we can relax, or so we're told and sold. There is a solution to what ails us, a cure for our emotional fatigue.

Evolution of a Self-Care Industry

What we now warmly refer to as *self-care* is in fact an $11 billion industry, and one that's been commodified by almost every other consumer industry imaginable: spa, bath, water, skin care, candle, wine, essential oil, flowers, travel, food, home design—you name it, they've all got a stake in the self-care market. In one 2020 study, *self-care* actually came up as the most-Googled search term of the year.[2]

But how did we get here, to this model of self-care? To understand better, let's step back and trace a bit of the history of this movement, this behemoth we call self-care. What was self-care before it became associated with spa treatments and retail therapy?

As far back as the fifth century, Socrates talked about the importance of *knowing thyself*. He encouraged his students to pay attention to their own thoughts, attitudes, and experience. An unexamined life, according to Socrates, was not worth living. It could be argued, and indeed was argued by the French philosopher Michel Foucault, that the practice of knowing oneself was the original form of self-care.[3]

Centuries after Socrates was teaching on a self-caring life, when our interest in ideal states of being had faded, self-care became more of a medical concept. In the 1960s and '70s, self-care was about creating autonomy and a better quality of life, primarily for the elderly and mentally ill. It focused on exercise and other healthy-living practices. In addition, self-care was targeted at post-surgery patients; it focused on teaching patients to take care of themselves so that their healing would be successful.

Self-care then morphed into something that was not just for patients, but also for health care workers, particularly those in high-risk and emotionally draining professions. Self-care started being talked about as something that people in caregiving professions needed for their own well-being, to avoid burnout and stress. Thus began the idea that we cannot take care of others if we are not okay, not just physically but emotionally as well.

In response to the civil rights and women's liberation movements, the self-care model took on yet another incarnation. It expanded beyond the individual and became attached to politics and power. Poor health was associated with poverty, and as such, health became the ingredient necessary to break down the power structure of race, gender, class, and sexual orientation. Inequity in health was seen as the most inhuman form of inequality. Nothing could happen, therefore, no power structure could shift, if everyone didn't have the chance to be healthy.

During these movements, self-care then became a form of protest, a way to empower a population and counter the injustice in our society.[4]

Yet another shift came in the latter part of the twentieth century, when self-care started being used in the context of wellness as an expansion on the traditional Western medical model. The idea was that we needed a more holistic attitude toward the human body and mind. Through self-care, we could proactively create our own well-being, as opposed to just going to doctors who treat disease. Wellness and self-care were then inextricably linked.

It was at that point that self-care took on a different tone, lighter and more positive than it previously had been. Fitness became a form of self-care that regular people took part in; health clubs proliferated, and the eastern practice of yoga started to appear in everyday lives. Wellness centers became part of the corporate structures, as self-care was seen as increasingly important for employee health and productivity.

And then 9/11 happened. The term *PTSD*, post-traumatic stress disorder, then became a mainstream part of our cultural dialogue. While mental health care workers had certainly been addressing the condition for a long time, primarily with soldiers returning from war, after the twin towers came down, PTSD arrived on the scene with an intensity and significance that was unprecedented. Self-care became a mandatory practice for those in the caretaking professions: trauma workers, first responders, social workers, and all the rest. Self-care was seen as a required practice for preventing the compassion-fatigue and emotional burnout that came from taking care of other people.[5]

Now, as we move further into the twenty-first century and technology proliferates, our values are changing. Our lives are increasingly focused on being productive—and, of course, generating wealth in the process. Self-care is keeping up with the times and promising to do just that: make us more productive. An employee practicing self-care will be a better employee and thus generate more wealth.

Our lives are increasingly focused on acquiring new products and experiences—buying whatever we think will make us feel better and happy. Self-care now comes with a promise, albeit unspoken, that if we do and buy enough of it, we'll end up not just peaceful and rejuvenated, but more importantly, with an abundant and good life.

Self-Care Is Not Working

Today we have billions of dollars' worth of products and services to choose from, all designed to take care of us and make us well. And we're purchasing these products and practicing these services at an unprecedented rate. Yet we're still stressed out and exhausted, maybe more than ever. We're buying well-being but our beings are unwell. What gives? What's wrong with this model? Why isn't self-care taking care of us?

In truth, there's nothing wrong with self-care or what it prescribes; who can argue with a chocolate facial or lavender candle? Bubble baths help far more than they hurt. There's nothing wrong with *us* and the way we're practicing our current model of self-care. What's wrong is that our self-care system, as superficially satisfying and temporarily soothing as it is, is simply the wrong remedy for what ails us.

But self-care is not just an inadequate and inappropriate remedy; if the problem were just that, it would be no big deal. The larger problem, the big deal, is that self-care in the way we're doing it is actually solidifying our emotional exhaustion, the very thing it's claiming to heal.

Another Chance to Should on Ourselves

To begin with, self-care has become another *should* on our to-do list, another potential shortcoming with which to shame ourselves. *Are you taking proper care of yourself? Are you—really—doing enough for yourself?*

And *If you're not, you should be.* This is what we continually hear from other people and in our own head. Self-care has become another responsibility to fulfill in order to become better versions of ourselves. It's another way to successfully prove that we care about ourselves. Ironically, women now have the additional burden of *owing* self-care to those who care about us and to ourselves. And if we're not doing it well enough, once again, we have no one to blame but ourselves.

Self-care, simultaneously, has become a mental concept, an idea that's disconnected from us and from our intuitive self-caring nature. Self-care, the concept, now dangles out there on its own, untethered from its organic source: *you.* If you go for a run because you want to feel your body moving, experience the feel-good endorphins that will come from exercising, it has a different effect than if you do it because you *should* or because you *know* it's good for you. For one thing, you're far more likely to get out the door if you're motivated by your own wanting rather than some idea of what the run signifies or *says* about you. The idea that you *should* run likely leaves you on the couch with your sneakers still in the closet. But even if you do get out the door, your self-care ends up being another task you check off your to-do list, and one that confirms your identity as a responsible woman who takes proper care of herself.

Strangely, the more self-care gains in popularity, the more it simultaneously loses its connection to the self it's meant to serve. We have effectively turned over our own self-care, outsourced it to more reliable experts who will gladly tell us how to care for ourselves. And we, dutifully, follow their wisdom. In the process, our most basic intuition, our deepest knowing, is interrupted—the drive to take care of ourselves and the wisdom to know how—without which, true self-care cannot be true.

There's another *should* that's gotten tangled up in our current relationship with self-care too, which further complicates our ability to receive what we need. In short, we're convinced that the wellness memes, essential oil diffusers, yuzu teas, and oxygen cocktails we're buying and ingesting by the truckload *should* make us well. If we're not satisfied and replenished from being swaddled in a cashmere blanket after a berry-infused facial, then there must be something wrong with *us*. Sadly, self-care has become another way for us to not be enough and to be guilty for not being able to receive what we need from what we're being offered.

But we're not satisfied by the self-care practices we're investing in for the simple reason that they're not the right ones to satisfy our real needs or nourish us at the roots of our exhaustion. Still, we keep believing and behaving as if they *are* what we need—as if the empress is actually wearing clothes.

Staying Distracted

Most self-care strategies provide short-term symptom relief and surface solutions to what are systemic problems. And yes, you feel good when you're soaking in a bubble bath; your muscles relax and your mind may float away to a distant land, far from the worries of the day. You may even feel good about yourself and get a boost from having done something *good* for yourself. But soon enough, you're exhausted…again.

But because the relief is temporary, we keep coming back for more: more advice, more products, more programs, more solutions from the experts who know what we need better than we know. Indeed, our entire self-care system relies on our chasing answers and staying distracted from what we don't want to feel and yet keep trying to fix.

Addictions, whether it's to alcohol, drugs, sex, shopping, exercise, or whatever else, allow us to temporarily avoid real issues. So too, our self-help strategies make us feel good for a little while so that we can forget about what's not working in our life.

While self-help's short-term relief won't harm us like addictions will, when it comes to addressing the deeper problems we face in relation to our own needs, these solutions are not only ill-equipped for the job they've been assigned, but they actually divert our attention from the deeper disconnection we feel; they keep us waylaid, with the equivalent of a pleasurable buzz. Ultimately, this self-care system keeps us soothed—pampered and busy, but light years away from what we really need.

The Endless Search

There is yet another problem with our consumerized self-care system. Namely, self-care is something we buy and do, an object or experience with which we supplement our life—an *add-on* to ourselves. The drawback with this premise is that, once again, it keeps you in the mode of searching, always looking for something outside yourself to fill what you imagine is missing on the inside, to satisfy your unnameable deficiency. With the unending and ever-fresh supply of products and services that promise to take care of you (and thereby complete you), you're always just one strawberry-scented loofah away from feeling the way you want to feel. If you haven't found that right teacher, class, body treatment, flower remedy, or essential oil yet, it just means you need to keep looking.

In all the searching and seeking, we strengthen the belief that, as we are, we're missing whatever it is we need to be whole and content. And simultaneously, that someone else is the expert on what we need, even when the subject is us. But no matter how unsatisfying, temporary, and ill-fitting the answers we find may be, still we keep searching everywhere for what we need—everywhere, that is, but inside ourselves.

When you believe that your foundational well-being relies on something external, your attention is perpetually focused outward—trying to find that magic fix. As a consequence, you stop experiencing yourself as a destination. You become—solely—a place of departure. And that's just what you do—depart from yourself.

This outside-in mindset, which you're schooled in from the time you're born, ultimately disconnects and alienates you from your own intuition, your inborn knowing. And thus, from your most reliable guide. In an attempt to take care of yourself, you abdicate your authority as the one who knows what's best for you.

Herein lies the subtler and more insidious consequence of the current self-care system: the fact that it keeps you endlessly seeking an authority outside yourself and thus turning away from and rejecting your own inner authority. The result is that you—and all of us together—are left feeling insecure and cut off from your own wisdom and truth. We don't trust ourselves and don't trust that if we stopped consulting everyone else on what we need, we might actually be able to take care of ourselves.

The Ultimate Self-Improvement Project: You

When you really think about it, the basic assumption of self-care is ludicrous. Namely, that it's reasonable to have to remind ourselves to be kind—to ourselves. And equally absurd, that it's acceptable to have to tell ourselves that we deserve our own attention. We've created a system in which our own self-care requires a sticky note to remember, and an entire industry to instruct us on how to execute. Remarkably, we're all on board with this. But in fact, there's nothing reasonable or acceptable about having to be convinced that we're deserving of care. Or that the most fundamental aspect of self-care—caring about ourselves—has been removed as the primary driver in the self-care process and handed off to an industry.

For some, self-care is simply about getting eight hours of sleep and taking a multivitamin. But for so many women, when we talk about self-care, what we're really talking about is self-improvement. We should initiate all these self-caring projects, not just because they make us feel good, but because they will make us *better* versions of ourselves. Remember the likability cage from chapter 1? If you look closely, even self-care contributes to its solidity and operating truths.

Self-care products and services are marketed as gifts to yourself, but below the marketing is a subtler message reminding you that you can never rest, never get comfortable in your own skin, and never allow yourself to be who you are right now. Rest assured, there's always more work to be done—on you—before it's okay to be who you are, or just *be* period.

From a young age, we women learn to initiate and navigate what will be an unending journey of self-improvement. It's for our own sake that we keep improving; why wouldn't we want to become better versions of ourselves? If we stopped trying to be better, we would be letting ourselves and everyone else down, failing at becoming our *best self,* which is code for *not this self.* Being alive, for a woman, means striving to improve who we are. Self-care, at a not-so-subtle level, is a smarter, sweeter-smelling, and more-empowered-appearing replay of an old message.

The Remedy for Reality

But the unspoken promise of self-care, really, is that if you do enough of it and take really, really good care of yourself, then you'll be guaranteed a good life. And here's the kicker...a good life where nothing bad happens to you. The subtle suggestion in self-care is that it will protect you from suffering. In this way, self-care is intertwined with the cultural conviction that life shouldn't be hard—at least not if we're doing it right.

But here's where the train goes off the rails, because life *is* hard and always includes difficulty. No one makes it out of here alive, no matter how many soothing honey baths she soaks in. No one makes it through life without great challenges and losses. The self-care wagon has gotten mistakenly hitched to the fantasy of a smooth ride through life and the belief that life should feel like cashmere, look like a celebrity social media post, and smell like fresh-baked bread. Unfortunately, while self-care rituals are often pleasurable and sometimes even powerful, while they can temporarily soothe us, they won't take away the deep wounds that life inflicts, and they most certainly won't win in a fight with reality.

But the fact is, sometimes we *are* nourished by an external activity or treatment. The beneficial effects may wear off quickly, which keeps us coming back for more, and yet the relief we feel is telling and reveals a lot about women's needs. The next chapter answers these questions: What does self-care provide when it *is* successful? What is the actual nourishment in nourishing self-care?

By understanding what heals our exhaustion, we can better understand the exhaustion itself. Furthermore, we can build a new self-care system that targets its root causes and offers women real and sustainable relief and replenishment, without the need for all the potions and lotions.

6

SELF-CARE AS A DOORWAY TO OUR DEEPER NEEDS

The self-care industry is problematic by design, this much is obvious. And yet, it's worth examining the particular forms of *outside-in* self-care that *are* effective. By *outside-in*, I'm referring to any treatment or experience that comes from an outside source and is something we cannot provide for ourselves. Massage therapy is often cited as one of those effective and healing forms of external self-care, which is why I chose to study it, and why I interviewed dozens of women about their experience of being "*on the table.*"

To be clear, I'm not recommending massage (or any other treatment), and I also recognize that massage is not available to many people because of its cost. Rather, I am simply using the efficacy of the massage experience as a doorway to examine what we *really* want and need—on the inside—and what we ultimately must be able to offer to and from ourselves. I've broken down what happens during a massage to better understand the actual nourishment we're seeking.

If body work isn't your thing, imagine a form of self-care that *works* for you and gives you just what you need. The point is not *what* the particular form is, but what it offers you that makes you feel taken care of and *fed*.

Dissecting a Massage: Reflections from Women on the Table

The massage therapist begins by simply placing her hands on our body. Still in busy mind, we may wonder when she is actually going to *start* the massage, or how much this *doing nothing* is costing us. Soon, though, the thoughts fade and we become aware of her hands and the dance of bodily sensations happening inside us. Our attention drops below the neck and in response, our body exhales—on its own—without our having to tell it to. Before our muscles have even been addressed, we may already feel better; we may already feel taken care of.

And then she begins to apply pressure, thoughtfully and without rushing—without our having to ask. During that time, we allow ourselves to experience the direct sensations, to be present inside ourselves, without trying to make sense of what's happening or why.

We may, at some point, find ourselves slipping back into old habits: breaking the silence we're deeply enjoying, redirecting the attention, and *leaving* ourselves, to offer feedback on what the therapist is doing so as to give *her* a positive experience—to take care of *her*. In other words, we may do what we're trained to do. But hopefully, we catch ourselves, get quiet again, and remember that this moment is for *us* and we are there to receive—*just* receive. If we can and do return to our own experience, we may receive real relief, not just for our body, but for our mind, spirit, and whole being. As a result, we may leave the room feeling genuinely taken care of and with the sense that our needs have been met.

And so, this begs the question: What happens in that experience that's so powerful—what *really* nourishes us? The body work is delicious, but what's the real nectar and sustenance beneath the physical relief? As it turns out, there are a multitude of restorative elements, consistent ones, in just about all of the experiences that genuinely take care of us.

Beyond the Ahhh of It

The invitation to be where we are. What comes up again and again in conversations with women is a strong wish and need to *get out of our head*—to figuratively *lose our minds.* Replenishing self-care offers the opportunity to do just that—to shift our attention from the busy mind of thinking, planning, managing, figuring out, and getting things done, and drop into the world of direct sensation. Self-care that *works* provides us with entry into this present moment; it allows us to shift from thinking about the past and future, to being here now. In essence, to move from thinking *about* our life to directly experiencing it.

In such moments, we have a chance to just stop—stop the running, accomplishing, and doing that we habitually do. We have permission to get off the hamster wheel of productivity, to be where we are and *just* where we are—without having to make anything else, more, or better happen. And as it turns out, it's not *more* that we need and crave in our lives—it's *less.*

A rare silence. In addition to this need for a break from all the thinking and doing, women express an appreciation (and longing) for silence. The wish, as it's often voiced, is to *not* have to engage in and *not* be bombarded by the cacophony of mental content and noise with which we normally contend. With silence comes a deep sense of relief, and restoration. Mind, body, and soul soak in the silence like water after a desert trek.

And indeed, the silence we experience often transforms from the absence of sound to a sound of its own, one that our whole being wants to listen to and rest in. Long after the silence has ended, we may still feel in touch with it. We might even start noticing the silences between sounds, which helps continue our process of replenishment. For so many of us, this simplest of experiences—quiet—is profoundly healing and exactly what our bodies, hearts, and minds crave. As such, it is an important (and often overlooked) element in what we need to recover from our exhaustion and what restores us to vitality.

Our own attention. The opportunity to be attended to by another human being is a remarkable experience. But what's even more remarkable is the chance to attend to ourselves, to have permission to possess our *own* undivided attention—to be *with* ourselves—without distraction or guilt. In successful self-care, we are offered this invitation—to settle into our own company and feed ourselves with our own undivided attention. This chance to come home to ourselves, and be free from having to take care of anyone or anything else, for most women is a rare and powerful occurrence.

A time to receive. At the heart of all successful self-care, no matter its form, is the opportunity to receive. And more specifically, to receive without feeling like we also have to give. Self-care that works provides us with the occasion to be *off-duty* as far as other people's needs are concerned. It's an invitation to experience something that's entirely *for us.* The root of all spiritual and emotional replenishment—its irreplaceable ingredient—is this profound experience of receiving. As obvious as it sounds, it bears stating and restating: in order to feel taken care of, we have to allow ourselves to *receive* care.

What we really want. The most powerful ingredient in nourishing self-care may, however, be its simplest: it gives us what we need because we actually *want* it. Self-care works (when it works) because we don't have to convince ourselves of its value…to reframe, contextualize, or assign a greater purpose to the act of self-care so that we can *want* to do it. It doesn't require us to engage in any mental gymnastics, to work at turning it into something that would be good for us or anyone else. Ultimately, we don't need to be convinced by our own mind that it's what we should want. So much of what we do as women is motivated by a sense of *should*. But in this case, the experience, the self-care, originates from a clear and direct *wanting*; it's inarguable and bigger than just an idea, responsibility, or demand—bigger than *us*, in fact. The wanting moves us, rather than the other way around. This experience is so powerfully replenishing precisely because it *is* so different than most everything else we do; we do it because we actually *want* to do it.

Peeling back the layers, it becomes clear that successful self-care provides us with an opportunity to experience something we genuinely need at a deep level, a need which is often hidden even to ourselves. And furthermore, that the fundamental components that make certain practices feel so self-caring turn out to be surprisingly consistent. We are restored physically, mentally, emotionally, and spiritually for a myriad of reasons that are in fact shared. Reasons that ultimately teach us what we must pay attention to and take care of inside ourselves.

You Don't Need the Spa, You Need You

Once again, I'm not here to sell you on massage or any other treatment, or to suggest that you need to put anything else on your *to-do* list. (Google can help you with that.) As enjoyable and sometimes helpful as some forms of *outside-in* self-care may be, if you really want to heal your exhaustion, to find a substantive and sustainable solution for your emotional depletion, you cannot rely on massages or any other outside experience, person, or product for your well-being. Real self-care is an *inside-out* practice; it's about being able to take care of yourself on a daily basis, in your regular life, without all the props and pampering we add to that life. You can still engage in all the props and pampering—why not?—but don't imagine them as the real answer to your depletion. Ultimately, self-care must be something that you can reliably offer to yourself; it must originate from inside of you. At the end of the day (and beginning and middle too), self-care is *not* an activity or thing, but rather a relationship you build and nurture with yourself.

If there's one thing self-care hinges on, it's this: a willingness to be with yourself in a friendly and accepting manner—to actually *be* self-caring. In order to get what you really need, you have to reframe the whole way you've been taught to relate to your needs and to yourself. Massages are wonderful, but what's even more wonderful is to realize that you contain everything you need for the creation of your own vitality, even when the spa is closed. All of the essential ingredients for true self-care already exist inside you.

Pay Attention to Your Habits—and Yourself

Before you can become your own caretaker, you must first become aware of how you are *not* acting as your own caretaker. If you want to live differently going forward, you have to start by living differently *now*, which means waking up to your current behaviors and patterns. Start by paying attention to your own attention; notice how you habitually give it away. Remember, what you give your attention to is what you're saying matters, imbuing with value, and awarding with power.

Our attention, as women, is perpetually on other people, wondering and fretting over *their* well-being, paying attention to how they are *with us* rather than how we are with ourselves. Our conditioning has taught us that our attention belongs to everyone and everything, with one caveat: everyone and everything but ourselves. To pay attention to ourselves is to say that we also matter, which is to be selfish.

But, once you can see this habit, you can then redirect your outwardly focused, inwardly abandoned way of operating in the world. With awareness, you can reset your conditioned patterns so that your own experience is *also* deserving of attention—and actually starts *receiving* your attention.

Paying attention to yourself may sound self-indulgent, pointless, or just plain wrong. Nonetheless, it's necessary. Nothing new can happen, no new relationship with yourself or the world, and no real self-care, until you claim your most basic right—the right to be interested in and attend to yourself—without guilt or shame. When you choose yourself as the destination for your own attention, you become the trustee of your own sustenance and the caretaker of your own needs.

Stop Tasking and Start Dropping—into You

Women are chronic multitaskers, for good reason. Most of us are responsible for taking care of what often feels like too much. We're forever thinking about who else needs our attention, what else needs to get done, and where else we need to be. We operate on the assumption that we can't possibly be *just* where we are, in *just* this present moment, with our attention *just* here. Not, that is, if we're going to successfully take care of everything else that needs taking care of. And yet this belief is not only false, but precisely the idea that renders us in a constant state of exhaustion.

If you're always tending to other responsibilities (even if it's just in your head), unable to let yourself *be* where you are, you remain chronically depleted. If you want to heal your exhaustion at a deep level, you have to give yourself permission to land in one place: here, now. To *stop* planning, managing, caretaking, providing, and what is essentially working all the time. You are rejuvenated when you let yourself be where you are—*just* where you are. And furthermore, when you trust that, contrary to everything you've ever been taught, the best way to take care of *everything else* is to take care of *this* moment right now, and maybe most importantly, to take care of the *you* who's living it.

Once you get the hang of paying attention to your own attention and redirecting it back to yourself and your own experience—what I call *bringing it home*—you are then in possession of a new superpower. At any moment, you can take a break from the internal chatter and busyness of your mind, and unhook your attention from the mental work of keeping everyone else okay. In so doing, you can nourish yourself with your own attention and presence. Whenever you want or need, you can choose to *stop and drop,* to make the shift from a human doing to a human being.

Self-care from the inside out demands that you start consciously pausing—not just physically, but mentally and emotionally too. And, that you take respites from attending to all that you attend to. It means learning how to let your mind be off duty. Just by dropping out of your head and into your body, taking one conscious breath, feeling your physical presence, you're *heading* in the right direction: *away* from your head. This simple choice, to shift from an external, *doing* focus to an internal, *being* one—to intentionally get still, go inside, experience yourself here in the present moment—is a profound act of restoring and recharging yourself. Just this *is* self-care.

Feel the Wanting

The reality is, playing all the roles we play, twisting ourselves into all the shapes we twist ourselves into, comes at a heavy cost. The cost, specifically, is that we stop listening to and recognizing the feel of our own *wanting*. We don't hear our *I want* when it whispers to us, sense it when it aches on our behalf, or respond to it when it screams. We learn to pay attention, exclusively, to the loud and trusted voice of *should* in our head; we're well aware of (and in constant contact with) what we *should* do and feel at any given moment.

Your conditioning has taught you to value the voice of *should* above all else. But real self-care requires that you start shifting the balance and tuning in, *not* to your inner *should-er*, but to the less mental and more sensorial energy of your inner *want-er*. It means consciously listening for the sound of I *want* inside you *and sensing for its unique perfume*. It requires recognizing and building a healthy respect and curiosity for the energy of *yes* that emanates from you. Replenishment, at the core level, demands that you build a new relationship with your own yearning—the yearning that, even after you've talked yourself out of it, still yearns. The voice of should, if you keep following it, will keep leading you to exhaustion. But *wanting*, if you have the courage to feel it and follow it, will lead you to the source of your fire, and ultimately, to what is most authentic in you.

Know, too, that the specifics of *what* you want are not important; committing to your own wanting is not the same as giving yourself the objects you desire. That may or may not come as a result. The process I'm describing is one of becoming aware of and befriending the experience of *wanting* in you, as it is own entity, which can mean simply getting in the habit of asking yourself what you want, noticing wanting when it arises, and acknowledging it when it shows up.

But ultimately, it means moving past the objects of wanting and into the source of it, the place from which the wanting itself emanates. When you can go there, to the place in you that wants; when you can know yourself there, gain access to that wisdom, then you are home. Then you have the keys to your own castle.

My Needs—Whose Job?

Most of us believe, at least at some level, that it's someone else's responsibility to figure out our needs—and not just figure them out, but also satisfy them. But in reality, if you're no longer a child, then that responsibility, that privilege, is yours and, to some degree, yours alone. This is not to suggest that your needs won't be taken care of by others. They will be, at times. But contrary to what you perhaps wish were true, and certainly the fantasy you've been sold, it's no one else's mandate—not your partner's, friends', family's, employer's, or anyone else's—to intuit your needs, nor to fulfill them (or to fulfill you, for that matter). It's lovely when it happens, but the task of taking care of and sustaining yourself ultimately belongs to you. When you take on this responsibility wholeheartedly, without resistance or resentment and without imagining it should be otherwise, then you are ready to live self-care in its most mature incarnation.

Most self-care strategies focus on action: what you need to do, how you need to advocate for yourself and behave differently in the world—so that you can get your needs met. Action is good and, of course, necessary. But to go straight to action, to start *doing* self-care before *being* self-caring, is skipping a fundamental and unskippable step. Until you change who you are on the inside, you're just practicing self-care-light; you're taking sound baths and buying yourself flowers when you don't yet care about yourself. It's moving straight to the outside experience and bypassing the inner experience. I, for one, don't want you to skip the step of caring about yourself.

The business of getting what you need is an inside job. In reality, you cannot relate differently to the world until you've learned (and are willing) to relate differently to yourself. It's not possible to be your own advocate until you've developed a heartfelt respect and affection for the you you're advocating for. Simply put, you can't get what you need from the world until you can get what you need from yourself. The chapters that follow are a recipe for just that.

7

A CARING RELATIONSHIP
WITH ALL OF YOU

Nicki's life was enviable to a lot of people; she adored her husband and three children, and had devoted her life to taking care of them and creating a wonderful home and family. And she'd succeeded at making that happen. Nicki was incredibly grateful for all that she had, and at the same time, she was in my office because she also felt caged and confused, and increasingly unsatisfied with her life. She hungered for something beyond domestic sweetness—to experience herself as more than just someone whose life revolved around other people and keeping them happy, no matter how much she loved and was devoted to those other people. She wanted to remember what it felt like to be fully herself, fully alive, and to find the woman who had disappeared into all her caretaking responsibilities. Nicki wanted a life that included who she was for real—not just who she was for everyone else.

Twinges of these longings had been appearing for years. But the twinges were getting sharper and more frequent. Still, each time her longing made itself known, Nicki went on the attack—self-attack. She angrily reminded herself that she had what everyone else wanted and was "unimaginably privileged." She was living a perfect life, so how dare she need what she needed? *What was wrong with her; how could she possibly be unsatisfied given all of her blessings?* The only answer was for her to stop feeling the way she felt, stop all her inner complaining, and as she put it, "stop the nonsense." Her feelings made her a bad person, and consequently, those feelings had to be eliminated. Unfortunately, as is always the case, when she eliminated her feelings, she also eliminated herself, which became the larger problem.

Like Nicki, you may remind yourself regularly that there's no good reason for you to feel the way you feel and no reason to need what you need. Allowing yourself to acknowledge your dissatisfaction, to listen to your own yearnings, would just make you feel worse about what you're not getting and worse about yourself.

But condemning your feelings doesn't help you feel better and certainly doesn't make the unwanted feelings go away. In fact, it makes the feelings grow stronger and inflicts more punishment on you—makes you the enemy—which further disconnects you from the self with whom you're aching to connect. The problem is that you're trying to find a way to take care of yourself without allowing yourself or your real needs to show up; you're offering self-care to a self that's not allowed to exist.

Eventually, Nicki turned to a different elimination strategy, and sadly, one that many women opt for when they've turned against themselves. It started with a glass of wine at dinner, but it wasn't long before she was drinking a bottle of chardonnay every day. She discovered, however, that the wine only numbed her feelings, and only temporarily. But those same feelings were still there, still unattended to, uncared for, and still demanding her attention. The boredom and stuckness remained, and the same wanting burned in her belly. In fact, when she wasn't anesthetized by the alcohol, the pain was even sharper.

After nearly two years of practicing this strategy, trying not to feel what she didn't want to feel and trying not to be the person she thought she would be if she didn't stay numb, it wasn't just her heart that was aching, it was her liver too. And so, thankfully, Nicki had the awareness and strength to change directions.

She turned to the self-care industry, which then became the new strategy—the new addiction. She invested in a high-tech light box, started a crystal collection, and learned to bake, do yoga, and take nature walks. She adopted a vegan diet, added Himalayan salts to her bath, and drank enough lemon water to sink the *Titanic*. She was convinced that the answer to her unwanted feelings, her unfulfilled needs, was to become a self-care devotee, a junkie of the self-care industry. In her words, "to finally make myself a priority"—in all the ways the industry suggested.

But unfortunately, just as chardonnay fails to solve real problems, self-care of this sort doesn't give you what you really need. It doesn't make the feelings you don't want (and are not supposed to have) go away. After doing everything possible to eliminate your emotional hunger, it's still there, still ravenous, and you're still to blame for being hungry.

The roots of our depletion are *not* in our life situations, even though our situations can be dreadfully difficult. Our exhaustion, rather, is more often a result of the punishing attitude we employ toward our experience and our feelings. We're depleted because of how we've learned to relate to ourselves *within* our difficult life situations.

Consider your own life: Are you dismissive and critical of your feelings? Do you judge your experience as the *wrong* experience to be having? Like Nicki, are you longing to connect with yourself, to be fully authentic, but also frustrated and disappointed by yourself and what you authentically feel?

It's an impossible predicament that leaves you in a battle not just with reality, but with yourself, and results in a state of unrelenting emotional fatigue. Once again, the real challenge you face has to do with your relationship with yourself.

The Keys: Awareness and Attitude

The two most important ingredients in potent and enduring self-care are awareness and attitude. Before anything can change, you must be willing to acknowledge what's happening inside your own mind, heart, and body. You must be ready to accept your reality *as* your reality, whether you want it as your reality or not. What's most important is that you generate an attitude of acceptance, of allowing *whatever* experience is arising within you—*whatever* truth is true. If you want to start taking care of yourself in a way that's truly replenishing and reliable, awareness and attitude are the two nonnegotiables in the process.

Learning to take care of yourself is not about tracking down some magic potion or unique experience, and not about finding a better system for getting rid of the wants and needs you think you shouldn't have. It is, more simply:

- Trusting that your experience cannot be anything other than what it is, that you are not to blame for your experience, and that your experience matters and is legitimate for the simple reason that it *is* your experience.

- Refusing to criticize, blame, or shame yourself for what you feel.

- Showing up for yourself—being willing to listen to, acknowledge, and unconditionally accept your own truth.

- Building a ground of self-kindness in which you are fundamentally and irrevocably on your own side.

What brought Nicki relief from her emotional exhaustion and what will bring you relief from yours is a shift in your relationship with yourself. You will discover fulfillment, paradoxically, from giving yourself permission to feel unfulfilled. You will unlock a sense of vitality from inviting in your own exhaustion. Over time, you will learn to acknowledge and empathize with your actual feelings—to stop judging and correcting your experience so that it can be what you think it should be. You will understand that you don't choose your feelings and aren't to blame for what you feel. The way you feel is the only way you can feel, and therefore, *has* to be okay. Ultimately, you will develop (as Nicki did) the nectar of self-care: namely, compassion and respect—for yourself.

Keep in mind, this change in Nicki's internal relationship didn't fix her domestic situation or make her life perfect. But it did change the way she related to and felt about her situation, and more importantly, the attitude with which she related to herself *within* that situation. In Nicki's old belief system, any difficulty or discomfort, any wanting, was proof that she had made bad choices in her life, and was, once again, at fault. But she came to understand that challenges, difficulties, disappointments, and wanting are just part of life, every human life, and that they coexist with all the things we cherish. Their existence didn't need to make her feel guilty or bad about herself or her choices. As a result, she discovered that she could appreciate her domestic life for what it offered, delight in its sweetness and her love for her family, and at the same time, acknowledge and empathize with her experience of what family life could not provide—what, for now, she would have to do without. With permission to stop shaming herself for her boredom and hating herself for wanting more, she could then offer herself kindness and understanding for the life choices she had made and the losses that accompanied them.

Nicki did something far more radical and far more self-caring than eliminating or *fixing* what was difficult in her life: She made friends with her truth, *all* of her truth, which included all of its contradictions. And in so doing, she made friends with *all* of herself.

The goal of self-care, or so we've been sold, is to remove what doesn't feel good and add what does. And yes, of course, this is a part of taking care of ourselves. But more often than we want or are willing to acknowledge, the truth is that we *can't* actually rid ourselves of what doesn't feel good, not because we're failing, but just because it's the way reality is.

Reality always includes a heck of a lot that doesn't feel good: situations and people that are imperfect (ourselves included), loss, and other challenges, which makes this *self-care as a difficulty-eraser* paradigm unworkable. Paradoxically, it's precisely when you're able to relax with what's difficult and to offer yourself kindness for your experience *within* the difficulty that you actually start to feel better—even radically better. This is the essence of real self-care—not *abolishing* the hard stuff but rather adding acceptance and compassion to it. With an internal attitude of *allowing what's true to be true*, you will discover that you can in fact make peace with your life in whatever form it's showing up. This shift offers a different kind of care from the sort you thought you needed. And indeed, it awakens a new buoyancy and well-being, for which, remarkably, *you* are the provenance.

So far, I've been defining self-care as the act of building a warm and welcoming relationship with yourself, nurturing an internal climate of acceptance and empathy, and giving yourself permission to feel whatever you feel. But there's one emotional experience that calls for its own conversation, one that's harder for women to acknowledge and relax with than any other—because it flies directly in the face of our female conditioning.

Anything but Anger

The message to women in our society is abundantly clear, even if the words are never directly spoken: Don't be angry; if you're angry and female, it's not okay and *you're* not okay. If anger is detected, there's a good chance you'll be dismissed as one of the following: crazy, aggressive, hysterical, irrational, hormonal, unattractive, nasty, bitter, harsh, unfeminine, hostile, and the all-time favorite, a bitch. Anger is a dangerous emotion to feel when you're a woman.

For the most part, women and men experience anger equally. But that's about all that women and men share when it comes to their relationship with anger. Boys are taught to view their anger as a sign of toughness; male anger moves the dial forward, is productive, and indicates power and confidence. Anger is considered appropriate for a man. When a man is angry, his character can remain intact in the face of his anger.

Girls, on the other hand, are taught that anger is inappropriate, shameful, and a sign of being out of control. We've failed if we've allowed ourselves to become angry. An angry woman is seen as less trustworthy, and thus is less likely to convince people of what she's angry about. When a woman is angry, the assumption is that there's something wrong with *her* rather than with whatever she's angry about. Her upset is evidence of her brokenness, which then removes not only the legitimacy of her grievance, but any need to address it.

So, from a very young age, we're taught to suppress our anger and figure out how to make it go away—which usually means changing ourselves. Anger conveys dissatisfaction, it means that we're not okay with the way things are; when our job is to *be okay*, anger doesn't exactly fit the bill. Welcoming our truth when our truth is anger, and at the same time, fulfilling our responsibility to be pleasing and make everyone happy, presents a difficult challenge. Anger isn't pleasing and doesn't generally make people happy. At the same time, being pleasing is in our best interest, or so we think. And so the answer is clear: we need to figure out a way to not be angry or at least not in touch with our anger.

Consequently, we've come up with all sorts of ways to manage our anger and prevent it from becoming threatening, not only to others, but to our own likability. When we can't pretend our anger doesn't exist, and can't behave as if everything is fine and we are fine…we have well-crafted strategies to keep ourselves in line.

Taking the High Road. One thing we women are really good at is taking the high road, rising above our anger, and being the *better person*. From the time we're old enough to recognize that other people exist, we're taught to take care of those other people, to be empathic and forgiving, and do what's best for everyone—not *just* ourselves. But unfortunately, not *just* ourselves is usually code for *not* ourselves at all. And indeed, we're highly praised for our willingness to sacrifice our needs and serve the collective and greater good. Our likability quotient goes up quickly when we put ourselves in other people's shoes and remove our own. As a reward, we may not get our real needs met, may not feel heard, seen, or relieved, but we do get to wear the badge of the noble and virtuous one. And we get to be liked and respected for keeping the peace, which goes a long way. The choice to take the high road is an admirable one; the problem is not that we do these things, but that we feel like we have to do these things.

Being Self-Deprecating. Another skill we've mastered as women is that of mocking and trivializing our anger, transforming it into something entertaining and, usually, self-deprecating. We laugh at our anger and ourselves, and in doing so, we make ourselves less threatening and more acceptable. But we also discredit and disown our own truth in the process. Our *not getting our needs met* becomes something that, ultimately, others can enjoy and get a giggle from, something that adds to our likability. Yet again, we trade what we want and need for being liked, which we believe is even more important.

Making It Tidy. When it comes to self-management for women, our long list of skills also includes a well-honed ability to wrap up our anger into reasonable and tidy packages, to make it rational, so that it can appear legitimate. We're masters at presenting our anger so that it makes sense, once we've thought it through and made it palatable, understandable, and, essentially, un-angry. But in doing so, we also drain our anger of its unpredictability and power, and consequently, its ability to create change for us—we drain ourselves of the constructive energy and possibility that anger contains.

Seeking Catharsis Elsewhere. Sometimes, however, we're not ready or willing to trivialize, sweeten, or wrap up our anger with a sensible bow. Nevertheless, we can still throw eggs at a wall, punch boxing bags, and scream into sound-absorbing pillows. If we must be angry, we can do it *positively*, without making anyone else uncomfortable or unhappy. We can be angry without anyone's having to hear or know about it; only the pillows and punching bags need suffer with our discontent. And yet, while temporarily cathartic perhaps, these physical releases are ineffective at taking care of the feelings and unmet needs that hide in the roots of our anger.

Boiled down, we've been conditioned to relate to our own anger as unfeminine, destructive, illegitimate, and a feeling that's not okay to claim—or as we like to say, *indulge*. Anger is a problem—*our* problem, and one that we're responsible for fixing.

And yet, we consistently ignore the fact that anger is an instinctively self-caring part of us. Our anger is here to protect us and alert us that we're *not* getting what we need and are not okay with what's happening. Anger is our discontent demanding to be heard and attended to, and refusing to agree with the party line that everything is fine and *we* are fine with everything. Tragically, we've been conditioned to turn away from our most natural self-protector and abandon the very feelings that are trying to take care of us.

Faced with the pressure and expectation to be endlessly pleasing, self-sacrificing, giving, likable, accommodating, appreciative, and always okay, anger is an unavoidable reality. We can't be all these qualities and also be authentic; we can't squeeze into the box society wants us to squeeze into without anger's being part of our experience. However, and here's where it gets tricky, anger is not supposed to be part of our experience; it's not on the list of acceptable emotions. And so, we're left at odds with our own reality. We are emotionally exhausted because we're continually tamping down, tucking away, and essentially waging war with a natural and necessary part of our experience, one that we can't *not* have, and yet one that we've been told is unacceptable and makes *us* unattractive.

Self-care, when it comes to anger, begins like everything else—with awareness. It begins by listening to and acknowledging your anger— without pathologizing it or yourself for its presence. It requires that you stop fearing your anger and treating it like the piranha society has convinced you it is. You've been taught that anger is dangerous, but in fact it is your ally, and most dangerous when you reject it and refuse it a seat at your inner table.

Interestingly, anger is a drive that, for the most part, is impervious to your conditioning. Anger has your back even when you've been taught to give your back away. Your anger defends you and knows you matter, even when *you* don't know it or won't allow yourself to know it. Anger rises up and shouts, *Hey you, stop. This is not okay.*

Remember too—underneath anger, there's always hurt; anger is the loud voice that speaks up for your quiet (or quieted) pain. In emotional language, anger is your heart and spirit saying, *No!* And underneath that *no*, there's an *Ouch...this hurts.* Regardless of what you tell yourself, anger breaks through and insists that you are worth defending. That said, your own anger is an invaluable mechanism in your emotional, spiritual, and physical well-being. Developing a healthy respect and curiosity toward it (which is not the same thing as acting it out) is a critical and too-often-ignored aspect of self-care.

You Need All of You

Real self-care must extend beyond your acceptable feelings, the ones you've been taught are okay to feel; it must include more than just those truths that are easy to acknowledge, safe, understandable, and most importantly, don't present a problem for anyone else. It demands building an accepting and respectful relationship with those parts of yourself that you think are ugly, embarrassing, mean, yucky, dangerous, and unlikable—the feelings that you thought made *you* ugly, embarrassing, mean, yucky, dangerous, and unlikable. To truly take care of yourself, you have to be willing to take care of *all* of you—the whole imperfect and messy enchilada. Nothing, not one want, need, feeling, or experience, can be deemed unworthy or excluded from your care.

The next time anger or any unwanted emotion arises, turn toward it, lean into it, ask it what it's angry or upset about, what it's not getting, what it needs to be okay—what *you* need. Once again, welcoming your truth does not mean acting it out, but rather inviting it in for tea, just as you would a cherished house guest. The truth is, your feelings are not going away; you may push them down, run from them, scold them into silence, anesthetize them with temporary pleasures, but they're still here, waiting for *you* to care about them.

I hope it's clear by now that self-care is *not* a thing or activity, but rather a relationship you build and nurture with yourself. In the next chapter, we'll switch gears and get our boots on the ground. We'll unpack what you need to learn and know (or perhaps unlearn and unknow) in order to start living this new relationship with yourself.

8

RECLAIMING YOURSELF

Patty came home to find her husband on the sofa watching television. Dinner had not been started despite his having been home from work for over an hour. When she asked if he had opened a bottle of wine, which was their ritual, he didn't answer, but just grunted something unintelligible. Interestingly, Patty did *not* ask her husband what was going on with him or why he hadn't started cooking, and did *not* share how ravenously hungry she was or how bothered she felt that nothing was on the stove.

Instead, Patty started fielding a deluge of thoughts about what she had said or done to cause her husband's bad mood. Perhaps she hadn't been as attentive to him lately as she normally was. Maybe she'd rejected an invitation to be intimate; is that what his hand on her back had been about? She wondered if the comment she'd made about his friends had upset him or sounded bitchy. The truth was, Patty had no idea what was causing her husband's strange and unfriendly behavior, but nonetheless, she was convinced of one thing: It was her fault. *His* bad behavior was because *she* had done something she shouldn't have done or had failed to do something she should have done. Case closed.

No matter what someone is experiencing—if it's not good—you probably assume, like many women, that you are the cause of it. Other people's feelings are *your* fault, a result of something you should have done differently. Even if you don't know how you failed and even if your intentions were good, still, you must have done something wrong. The habit is to personalize everything and make everything about your failings. Well, that's not entirely true…you probably don't make everything about you, just everything that needs to be fixed.

Let's look at how this played out for Marjorie…

Marjorie and her dear friend Pascal were enjoying a nice lunch together when Pascal began sharing something he'd read in the news, an issue that bothered him and on which he had a host of theories and strong opinions. Marjorie listened for a while and then shared her own thoughts on the topic, about which she also felt passionately and also knew a lot—a lot more, in fact, than Pascal.

As she was sharing, however, Pascal became noticeably quiet; he lowered his eyes and seemed to withdraw into himself. While he had been animated when sharing his own thoughts, now, with Marjorie taking part in the conversation, Pascal had stopped participating and also stopped listening. He had, in effect, left Marjorie alone to espouse her views into thin air.

Witnessing her friend's disappearance, Marjorie instantly felt guilty and ashamed. *Why do I have to be such an attention hog? Why did I need to steal his thunder? Why do I always have to be so pushy and steal the spotlight?* And the kicker, *Why am I so emasculating?* This is where Marjorie *went* with her friend's response to what was, essentially, her adding her voice to the conversation. In her internal narrative, she had inserted herself where she wasn't welcome, dominated Pascal, and forced him into submission. She was sure that it would be a long time before he found the courage and trusted her enough to put himself out there again, which was understandable given her unfeminine and aggressive behavior.

In her storyline, she had eviscerated this man and stamped out any chance for continued conversation or closeness. It was her fault that she now felt lonely and abandoned, her fault that she felt ashamed, and her fault too for *making* her friend feel insecure. In a nutshell, everything happening, including her upset, was her fault.

Healing the It's My Fault Default

Patty's and Marjorie's reactions may sound bizarre and extreme, but sadly they are common for women. If you see yourself even a little bit in either woman's response, the first thing you need to know is that you are *not* responsible for everyone else's experience. *Just because someone is not okay does not mean it's your fault, that you caused it, or that it's your responsibility to correct it.* If there's one truth you take away from this book, take *that* one. Reality, when it's not to your liking (or someone else's liking), is not a mandate for you to figure out what you did wrong. Healing your emotional exhaustion requires that you stop trying to figure out what you did wrong and stop assuming the blame for...well... everything.

We women are depleted in large part because we spend so much of our time and energy trying to figure out what we did wrong and how we can fix our presumed failure. But real self-care begins when figuring out our failings and correcting our presumed inadequacies are no longer our primary pursuits in life, and maybe even (dare I say it) no longer of particular interest to us. It begins when we give up the delusion that if we could just be better and do better, we could make everyone and everything okay.

Feeling empathy for someone's experience and assuming responsibility for fixing it are radically different things. It's not a package deal; you can feel empathy for someone's pain and still let their pain stand without feeling like you caused it or have to fix it. Even when your truth is the spark for painful feelings in another, still, you didn't *cause* their feelings in the way you're taught to think about it. Your truth and another person's experience of your truth can coexist without either needing to be fixed or eliminated.

We are so deeply ingrained with the belief that if someone is suffering, it's our job to rectify it. But if you are going to heal your emotional exhaustion, you have to surrender this assumption of responsibility and control and let go of this cause-and-effect movie playing in your head, in which you are the writer, director, and star of the show.

Your exhaustion will heal *not* when you succeed at making everyone happy and figuring out how to better control your life and everyone else's, but just the opposite—when you learn to let go of control and allow for difficulty to exist in other people, and even the people you care about. You'll feel replenished and your vitality will return when you stop working so hard to make life go the way you think it should go.

Moving out of the universal-fixer role also includes accepting your limitations when it comes to making everything the way you think it should be. Even if you wanted to correct the problems you see, you might not be able to. Plus, the people and situations you're *fixing* might not want to be fixed. And even more scandalously, you might not actually *want* to spend your energy on fixing them. You have to be able to discern if and when you *want* to address the problems you see—if and when they're worth your time, emotional energy, and the mental real estate they occupy. Your assumption of universal responsibility leaves you compulsively fixing, with no choice as to where your energy and attention are going. It leaves you exhausted, emotionally and in every other way, with nothing left for yourself.

But when you stop assuming that everything is your fault and responsibility to make right, you will likely discover that you have a lot more energy, not just for others, but also for yourself. You're free to care about what you actually care about instead of being compelled to care about everything and everyone. As a result, you feel more alive, more authentic with others, and more connected to yourself. You can then get curious about what really matters—to you.

Released from the universal-fixer role, remarkably, you also feel more genuine empathy. You can understand and feel other people's problems, separate from your obligation to fix them. Your desire to help, when it does arise, is more real and less obligatory; it comes from *want* not *should*. Most importantly, when you loosen your grip on making everything and everyone okay and are willing to let things be *not okay*, then you are free to see what's really happening—to be in reality as a free and unburdened participant.

From Self-Improvement to Self-Worth

Our readiness to take responsibility for whatever is wrong in the world is not just saved for the outside world, however—it applies equally, if not more rigorously, to ourselves. *How can I be better?* This is the central question and operating paradigm from which we live. On the surface, the question sounds like a healthy and important one, a contemplation that would encourage us to keep growing and evolving. *How can I be better?* It sounds like an inquiry that we would be remiss to abandon and also criticized for relinquishing. We imagine that the question, when relentlessly considered, prevents us from getting too comfortable with ourselves (which would be a dangerous thing). We have been conditioned to believe that if we stopped constantly posing this question to ourselves, and everyone else as well, we would be declaring ourselves a finished product and claiming that we no longer need to improve or change in any way.

In order to stop feeling so depleted, we must shift the basic intention from which we live. The drive to always be better, while revered in our society, is in fact counterproductive and disempowering. Our celebrated drive to improve actually fosters the belief that who we are *now* is not good enough, which keeps us from ever being able to land and stand in ourselves. We're always chasing some new and improved version of ourselves, always trying to become someone *else* who presumably will be good enough to value themselves. But in the meantime, we remain perpetually exhausted—in pursuit of someone who is not us.

Keep in mind, the decision to stop trying to become a better version of yourself does not imply that you consider yourself fully evolved or perfect. You're never fully evolved or perfect; no one is. But as your primary intention in life, self-improvement gets in the way of your evolution. As admirable as it sounds, and as many likability points as you'll earn for it, self-improvement is really code for self-correction. With self-improvement/self-correction as your driving force, you remain broken and inadequate, denied the right to inhabit yourself now, which, ironically, is the only place your *evolving* can actually happen. Your emotional exhaustion eases when you accept that, like it or not, life will continue teaching you what you need to learn and how you're required to grow; life will do that for you without your needing to ask. Relating to yourself as a self-improvement project is not only a distraction from who you are now, but also a compulsion that reinforces your insecurity, and therefore your exhaustion.

When you relinquish self-improvement as your primary purpose, you can start getting to know yourself for real. Without the constant pressure to improve, you can get interested in who and how you actually are now, not the fictional version of you that you'll become in an imaginary future. This shift, from focusing on who you need to become...to meeting who you actually are, is at the core of building an intimate and friendly relationship with yourself—and therefore, at the core of real self-care. I promise you that you will not stop growing, become conceited, or end up stunted if and when you let go of your obsession with self-improvement. In fact, letting go of the hope (and demand) of becoming someone else will be the first and most important step in becoming an authentic incarnation of who you are.

Learning to Toot Your Own Horn

After years of listening to women talk about themselves, I became aware of how frequently and rigorously we put ourselves down and how hard and seemingly dangerous it is for us to talk about ourselves in an unapologetically positive way. It became clear that learning to toot our own horns would be an important step in revitalizing ourselves.

Not surprisingly, I received some less-than-favorable reactions to this idea. Men often responded with a hesitancy that veered toward disapproval: "Hmm…that's interesting, but is that really what you think women need—to brag more?" "But Nancy, do you think a strong woman should have to *flaunt* her strength?" "So you want women to be more like men, is that the goal?" The suggestion that a woman would be so bold as to sing her own praises appeared to elicit not just uneasiness, but also judgment.

And yet, when I floated this same idea to women, for the most part, I received a very different reaction. Permission to speak highly of ourselves, to shine without feeling guilty or ashamed…just the thought of it was met with great enthusiasm. But many women also confessed that they didn't think it was possible—*not*, that is, without also being judged as arrogant, self-involved, and attention-seeking. "The selfless caretaker doesn't really line up with speaking highly of ourselves" was how one woman put it. And it's true; if we want to be selfless, liking ourselves out loud presents a problem.

When we acknowledge ourselves, others may assume that we need attention, or less kindly, we *desperately* need attention. And of course, that wanting or needing positive attention is a bad thing. In acknowledging ourselves, we are failing at being selfless and invisible. Wanting to be recognized is not just an unattractive quality, but also a sign of weakness, or so we've learned. It implies that we aren't humble or secure enough to be satisfied without recognition. Furthermore, if we're talking about ourselves positively, we're probably either conceited or exaggerating our strengths, or both. Understandably then, with all this negative judgment awaiting us, we rein in our natural and healthy need to appreciate ourselves. What's clear is that we don't toot our own horns without very carefully and vigilantly managing other people's experience of our *horns*. We get very good at *not* needing appreciation, and making sure that everyone knows we *don't* need or want it (even if we do). How shameful it would be if we actually wanted to be seen and valued, and how arrogant to suggest or assume that we actually deserve it.

But in fact, wanting to be seen and appreciated is a healthy and normal drive, one that exists in every human being. And yet, we buy into our conditioning and presume that, as women, our wish to be positively acknowledged is a failing—embarrassing, and something we shouldn't need.

Healing your exhaustion requires breaking out of these habitual self-deprecating and self-invisibilizing patterns; while they were originally created to protect you and keep you likable, they now contribute to your depletion. It's important to be able to talk about yourself with confidence and respect, no matter what story gets written about that choice. The sort of horn-tooting I'm suggesting has nothing to do with conceit or grandiosity. In the context of a self-caring life, tooting your own horn means being willing to acknowledge whatever wants and needs acknowledgment in you. And simultaneously, allowing yourself to admit that you respect and care about yourself, whatever it's for, or if it's for no reason at all—just because you do.

The more I examined the issue of emotional exhaustion, the more I wondered how it's possible that we spend so much time and energy trying to improve ourselves but we never get to arrive at a place of genuinely liking ourselves. Are we supposed to just keep searching, but never reach our destination, never arrive at being good enough? The only way to break free from these cultural patterns is to start recognizing them, challenging them, and acting in ways that actually break them.

When you speak positively of yourself and admit that you like yourself, you bolster your own belief that you matter. At the same time, you demonstrate that it's okay for a woman to want to be seen and appreciated. The more you acknowledge yourself, internally and externally, the more you learn to trust that you are indeed worth acknowledging. Naming and claiming your value and also refusing to buy into the myths about women who do so are empowering and self-nourishing practices—and one to start today, whether or not you feel ready.

Making Yourself a Destination

One of my favorite stories is of a wild gazelle who, early in her life, smells a scent so magnificent that she spends her entire life searching for it, driven by the longing to reexperience its beauty. Many years later, as she lies dying, with her flank torn open by a hunter's arrow, she's engulfed in the scent she'd spent her life pursuing and in the magnificence she'd always craved. The scent was coming from inside her; it was *her* perfume—*her* magnificence all along.

Everything about the way we live in this society is geared to pull our attention outward and away from ourselves. We rely on external sources for information, knowledge, belief systems, entertainment, physical subsistence, codes of behavior, and everything in between. At the same time, we're sold the idea that our happiness will also come from the outside: acquiring external validation, material possessions, achievements, and pleasurable experiences. Over time, we come to believe that everything desirable, satisfying, and fulfilling, everything we want and need, comes from outside of us. Our focus is so habituated to go outward, in fact, that we forget that we are even here and can be a source of anything. We forget—or maybe more accurately, never learn—that we can look to ourselves for what we need.

In order for self-care to take root as a way of living, you must be willing to consider that you know infinitely more than you've ever been allowed or allowed yourself to know. And furthermore, to recognize that you are the only one who knows what's true for you, the only one living your unique experience. In fact, while it's the last thing the self-care industry wants you to discover, *you* are your most reliable source of well-being, even if you can't imagine it yet.

But remember, the conditioning that led you to abandon yourself, to hand over your authority to others and the external world, didn't happen overnight. Similarly, reclaiming yourself as a valuable source of wisdom also doesn't happen overnight. Before you can live a new path, you must be able to see the path you're traveling now—all the ways you're turning away from your truth and handing off your authority. In order to create real change, you have to be willing to challenge your conditioning and practice new behaviors.

Just as you build the habit of exercising by actually exercising, you have to build the habit of making yourself a destination by doing just that: making yourself a destination. You have to be willing to look to yourself for answers—and questions too. To spend time inside yourself, getting curious about your own experience and actively caring about you—the same you who's been taught to care about everyone else *but* you.

With practice, the inclination to turn toward yourself for guidance becomes second nature. But again, it doesn't start out that way. The process of learning to trust yourself happens gradually. Over time, you'll likely start noticing that you feel more present, more *located* inside yourself, as if you're living from something solid that feels like *you*. Without trying, you'll find that you're speaking what's actually true and being honest rather than saying what will secure your being liked. You'll feel the gap closing between who you are and the roles you play in the world. I've heard the process described in many different ways, but what all of the descriptions have in common is a sense of taking your seat at the center of your life—coming home to yourself.

Keep inquiring into your own experience; keep spending time in your own company; keep tuning into your own presence. Over time, your outward-focused wiring will shift and your attention will start naturally returning home to you, its original source. And indeed, with intention and practice, you will become that destination, that magnificence, for which you've always been searching.

So far, we've been looking at the internal shifts needed to make self-care a part of who you are, but now let's turn our attention to the action part. How does inside-out self-care walk, talk, and relate to others; how does it show up in the world? The coming chapter is a guide for living self-care as a basic operating system, one that's integrated into who you are and no longer just an occasional one-off you give yourself because you *should*. A self-care approach that's about more than just keeping you safe and likable inside a system that keeps you exhausted.

9

TELLING YOUR TRUTH

Three days before Fiona's fortieth birthday, her partner, Larry, asked her what she wanted for a present. He then went on to explain that because of commitments at work, he hadn't been able to do any shopping yet. Also, that he'd started calling around for dinner reservations and she should know that every restaurant so far was booked. So, maybe they could just order in something nice for dinner instead.

Larry had asked her what she wanted while simultaneously letting her know that she probably wasn't going to get what she wanted. Fiona loved dining out, but her conditioning, maybe like yours, had taught her to make the situation work—whatever the situation is. The basic instruction is to *not* inconvenience anyone, nor ask for anything that requires effort.

Growing up female, it's ingrained in us...*Be a good girl...don't be a problem.* The benefits abound for behaving as we've been taught to behave, not the least of which is avoiding the criticisms that await us when we misbehave. If Fiona had been a *good girl*, she would have used that moment when she learned that Larry would not be doing anything special for her fortieth birthday—to take care of Larry. She would have made it okay that he had not planned anything. Being a *good girl* would have meant making Larry feel good about Larry, regardless of whether it felt good for Fiona.

Without missing a beat, Fiona showed me her *good girl, no-problem* self. "'Oh wow,'" she'd said sweetly, "'thanks for the thought. And yes, ordering in a special dinner would be great for my birthday...I know you're really busy, but if you do stumble on something you think I would like, whenever, then just get it then. It doesn't really matter when...' And if I'd really been on my game, I might have added, 'I appreciate it, but really, I don't need anything at all,' just to seal the deal."

But in this case, Fiona mustered the courage to *not* be a good girl and to tell her partner the truth, which she did with a straightforwardness that surprised even her. Without belittling her own wishes, calling herself high-maintenance, demanding, bossy, ungrateful, or any of the other readily available insults, and without making a big case for why she deserved what she wanted, she simply and directly said that she would love a gift on her birthday and would love for him to plan something for her. And she added, "That's what I want for my birthday," which was also true. What made this moment so powerful was its simplicity—what it didn't include, rather than what it did. Fiona let the truth stand on its own—unadorned and undoctored. She let the chips fall where they needed to fall in the face of her truth.

Sadly, this kind of honesty and clarity in relationships is hard and scary for many women, particularly when it comes to asking for something we perceive as inconvenient, difficult, or the biggest one of all, undeserved. We believe that telling our truth, when it doesn't line up with someone else's truth, is hurtful and aggressive—uncaring. And, that it will cost us our important relationships and endanger our loving bonds.

But yet again, this belief is false. We can be truthful; we can say no—with awareness and care—while maintaining connection. We just haven't learned that we *can* do it or how to do it. Telling our truth, in fact, is the beginning of real connection, and if practiced mindfully, can and will strengthen our loving bonds.

Fiona, in this instance, stated her truth without adding all the bells and whistles that would normally be added to make it something her partner would want, all the sweeteners that would go into success- fully managing his experience. With that one simple but bold sen- tence, she took a gigantic step forward and accomplished something profound in her own journey. And she knew it. As a result, no matter what happened on her birthday, Fiona felt proud of herself, alive, and most of all, real. In her words, "I gave myself the best birthday present imaginable—*myself.*"

Hanging Up Your Good Girl Shoes

When we follow Fiona's example and speak truthfully and unapolo- getically about our wants and needs, no matter how insignificant or trivial they may seem (there are no insignificant or trivial truths), we leave the likability cage behind. When we express discontent and allow ourselves to *not* be okay with what's being offered, we change who we are. Just this—for a woman to be able to say *no… No, I'm not okay with that,* and *No, that doesn't work for me,* or, simply *I want*—is positively transformative.

The second process Fiona models in this example is that of express- ing our truth and allowing others to respond to our truth in whatever way *they* need to respond. When we take ownership of our own experi- ence, our part of the interaction, and simultaneously surrender control of the results and the response, we free ourselves of the burden of having to be responsible for everyone else's experience. We step out of the role of emotional traffic controller and give the job of managing feelings back to those others to whom the feelings and the job belong.

Finally, in being forthright and unapologetic about what she wants, Fiona shows us a way to communicate that our experience matters, that our truth is valid, and that our needs are entitled to a seat at the table. And furthermore, that our needs are not something extra, special, or privileged that should require our *demanding*.

Larry made it clear to Fiona that her feelings were inconvenient for him. But even with her partner's bother, she was able to stay connected with her truth and grounded in her own experience, without taking on his feelings as her fault or responsibility. For many women, *this* self-alignment is nothing short of revolutionary.

Our truth can be difficult for others to hear and accept, and yet we can still stand in that truth without identifying as *the one* who is difficult, and *the one* who has caused the discomfort. We can hold onto a self-experience that's *clean*, and not defined by another's perceptions and how we're being received. By standing in the validity and dignity of our own experience, holding our truth right smack in the middle of another's discontent, we are standing up to the cultural narratives and projections that define us. (More on this later.) As Fiona so beautifully expressed, "Who knew that just saying I wanted a birthday present could be so exhilarating, and the best birthday present I could ever receive!"

Standing with Yourself

Self-care is about choosing to stay on your own side, to stay connected and loyal to your truth, and to do it again and again, even when it's hard, awkward, unpopular, and scary, and even when it feels like it would be so much easier and more comfortable to adjust, accommodate, and soften your truth—to make things go smoothly.

But chances are, you already know how to make things go smoothly and are quite good at it. And furthermore, while making things go smoothly at all cost may result in…well, smoothness, it also may result in making you feeling unknown, unreal, and unhappy. True self-care is not about making things easy or smooth; it is about *not* abandoning yourself, and choosing to travel the harder and sometimes bumpier road of *not* doing what you're conditioned to do. To stand and stay with yourself above all else.

"It was intoxicating," Astrid said, nearly breathless. "Honestly, I don't even know who said it, it felt like a different me!" This brilliant, beautiful fifty-one-year-old woman then explained how she'd just said no to the opportunity that a colleague had offered her. An opportunity that her colleague had been proud to present, but which, in Astrid's estimation, only benefited her colleague's career. The intoxicating part, as she explained, was not that she had turned it down, but how she had turned it down. "Rather than making sure he knew how grateful I was for the incredible chance (which it wasn't) that he was offering me, I just thanked him for thinking of me and told him, respectfully, that I wasn't interested and it wasn't the direction I was going in my career. I didn't apologize for not wanting the project or explain what was wrong with me that made me not want it. What I did do, however, was express myself clearly and honestly, say what I needed to say without *adding on* anything to make sure it was okay with him and that he was okay with me. I know it sounds tragic, but for the first time in my adult life, except maybe with really close friends, I shared what was actually true, without making sure it worked for everyone else."

What's radically different and exhilarating about Astrid's response is that, like Fiona, she doesn't jump through all the hoops we normally jump through, doesn't sugarcoat the truth with all the white lies we coat it in to make it taste good and go down smoothly. She says less rather than more, keeps her words simple and direct, and lets the truth stand for itself. In so doing, she chooses not to participate in the emotional obstacle course of trying *not* to appear ungrateful or entitled and *not* to make the other person feel disappointed while trying to make them feel appreciated and important—while never *letting on* that we have needs and an experience of our own or that we might have a different idea than theirs about what's good for us. Astrid demonstrates how we can stop working so hard and navigating all these hurdles in our efforts to get what we actually need.

The Courage to Ask

Hazel worked a day job, but on Thursday nights, she also worked as a singer in a club on the opposite side of town. At the end of the workday, she would rush from her office to the club, changing clothes and doing her makeup on the train. Because of the unpredictability of the Metro, however, she often had to go straight onstage without a warm-up when she arrived, and sometimes she didn't even make her set time. But Hazel had accepted the physical and mental stress that went with having two jobs; she understood and frequently reminded herself how lucky she was to get to do what she loved.

She'd been at the same company for close to a decade, and yet it had never occurred to Hazel to ask her employer if she could leave ten minutes early on Thursday evenings and maybe make up the ten minutes on another day. She had never made such a request because, as she told me, "It's not my employer's job to accommodate me." To ask for *special* treatment so that she could do what she loved to do would have been assuming that *she* was special and better than other people who didn't get that privilege, which was out of the question and embarrassing to even consider. Furthermore, a request for anyone to have to adjust to her and her needs made her feel like a burden to her coworkers, which was also out of the question.

As if all of that weren't enough, this small ask, in Hazel's mind, would have meant announcing that she required *extra* care, which would mean admitting that she was *weak*. Those ten minutes, even if she was going to give them back on another day, would have been an indication that she couldn't be the entirely self-sufficient woman she had always prided herself on being. It would have meant asking others for help, which felt not just weak, but also helpless. And so, Hazel had remained quiet for a long time and made it work, unwilling to risk the threat of being a bother.

But then something happened: Hazel discovered that an important music producer was coming to the club to hear her set. This was her dream. Understandably, she did not want to entrust her chance at being *discovered* to the reliability of the Metro. This opportunity meant everything to her, and she was unwilling to waste it. Her fierce and undeniable wanting gave her the courage to ask for what she needed, to risk being a bother and a burden—weak, helpless, and entitled, all of it. So, she told her boss matter-of-factly, reciting the script she had rehearsed dozens of times with friends and in her head, that she would have to leave ten minutes early on that particular day as she had an event for which she couldn't be late. Her boss nodded without asking any further questions, giving her only a curiously raised eyebrow in the process. And that was that.

While it may sound surprising that it would feel so dangerous for a successful, intelligent woman to ask for something so measly, and also strange that I would dedicate a whole section of this book to just saying what's true and asking for what we want, for many strong, smart, and accomplished women, saying what's true and asking for what we want and need is, in fact, often a Herculean challenge. We struggle mightily with the asks that are for and about ourselves, no matter how difficult *not* asking makes our life; we'll put up with a hell of a lot before we'll risk the ask. But we don't know another way...until we do.

For Hazel, like Fiona and Astrid, simply asking for what she actually needed without rationalizing, apologizing, or trying to control her manager's response to it was a life-changing event. Not only did it change her career (she got hired as a full-time singer), it changed *her*. In

Hazel's words, "It liberated me." Simultaneously, it showed her what it looked, sounded, and felt like to genuinely take care of herself, and consequently, *get* what she needed.

Let It Be Uncomfortable

From the time we're young, we're conditioned to believe that it's our job to keep other people happy. We're also steeped in the flip side of that belief: namely, that no one should have to exist in a state of discomfort or displeasure. We imagine such states to be intolerable. Intolerable, that is, for *other* people. Interestingly, though, we don't consider discomfort or displeasure intolerable conditions for ourselves. We can manage being not okay; we'll figure it out; we'll survive. But no one else should have to live through the experience of being uncomfortable. Even if they could tolerate it, we can't. As we see it, allowing someone to exist in a state of discomfort without immediately correcting it is uncaring and selfish...a failing on our part. If we allow it to happen, we're not doing our job as women.

Real self-care requires breaking free from your conditioning as it relates to the whole notion of discomfort. It means learning to allow other people's discomfort to exist, and to stop trying to protect everyone from feeling disappointed, mistaken, insecure, or anything else we deem unacceptable or unbearable. Just as *you* have the capacity to tolerate difficult feelings, others too have that capacity. This is very good news. You can trust that displeasure, dissatisfaction, discomfort, and all the other dis-conditions are in fact inhabitable and survivable states—and not just for you. You take care of yourself, paradoxically, when you let other people decide what *they* need to do to take care of themselves. Just as *you* learn, grow, and change in response to discomfort, so do other people—if you will let them.

At the risk of repeating myself, here goes: That you are not what someone else wants you to be does not mean that you have failed or failed them. That bad feelings happen does not mean that you've done something bad or that you are bad. Know this: When you are brave enough to tell the truth, share what you feel, need what you need, and also strong enough to allow other people to experience your truth in whatever way they need to experience it, without controlling it, then you have not only *not* failed, but you have triumphed as a woman in a most revolutionary way. When you put these steps into action, every day is your birthday, as you are literally birthing a new self.

But speaking the truth, like everything new and different, can trigger fear and anxiety; it's uncomfortable and unfamiliar. And yet, the more you stand in your truth—even *with* the fear and anxiety that it triggers—the easier and more natural it gets. Remarkably, when you're no longer expending all your emotional energy on softening and "nice-ifying" your truth and on everything else it takes to exist safely, smoothly, and likably, you're free to live as the *real* you.

Over time, this way of living authentically becomes less effort-full and deliberate, and also less frightening (I give you my word on that). Living from and *as* yourself soon becomes second nature and no longer something you have to manufacture. Indeed, it becomes something you won't believe you ever did have to manufacture. Ultimately, your truth, with practice, becomes inseparable from who you are and how you move through the world. As a result, you find yourself energized, rather than exhausted.

Being You Is Worth the Risk

As women, we've been taught to believe something abjectly false. Namely, that taking care of ourselves involves becoming what other people want us to be, which requires managing our authentic wants and needs and doing away with the parts of ourselves that don't fit into a likable package. The consequences of this self-shifting process have been overlooked, deemed irrelevant, or viewed as a necessary sacrifice to keep ourselves safe and happy.

But what happens to you through this process of becoming what's wanted *is* relevant, and it is in no way a necessary sacrifice for safety or happiness. What happens, to be specific, is that *you* go away...you abandon yourself in an effort to become what's wanted, which cannot possibly take care of you. Being accepted at the expense of being yourself, being liked while having to betray yourself to accomplish it, cannot possibly give any of us what we really need.

Taking care of yourself is something quite different than what you've been taught. Real self-care is not about figuring out how to be what's wanted. I'm going to say that again: Real self-care is not about figuring out how to be what's wanted. It is, however, about figuring out who you are and having the courage to trust your own experience and knowing. Self-care happens when your allegiance shifts from being liked to telling the truth, which may not be pleasing to everyone all the time. And that's okay. When you live with your truth as your touchstone and anchor, then you always have yourself on your side, which is worth more than all the likability you could ever muster.

Opportunities to tell the truth and ask for what you need appear every day in situations from the most trivial to the most profound. What's important is that you notice and seize these opportunities. You can start by taking small chances, like asking for more milk in your coffee than you were poured, saying *no* to an engagement you don't want to attend...and then work your way up to the bigger stuff, like what you need emotionally from your partner, friend, or anyone else.

Every truth you tell matters and is a step toward reclaiming your authenticity and reestablishing your connection with yourself. Every time you tell it like it is, step outside your comfort zone, risk being honest, and show up as you are, regardless of the content or context, you are actively refilling your emotional bucket—nourishing yourself. When your primary loyalty (and commitment) is to the truth and your deepest intention is to stay with and not abandon yourself, then a self-caring life is underway and your exhaustion is being healed.

10

WRITING YOUR OWN STORY

Gwen was a working comedian when I first met her. She wasn't famous yet, but it seemed that she was on her way there. She was an artist who pushed herself hard. No matter how bone-tired she was, she showed up at every audition and never turned down a potential opportunity. As she saw it, that one just might be *the* one that would launch her. When Gwen wasn't auditioning, networking, or exercising (to keep herself camera ready), she was writing material, making videos, and applying for jobs. Or, she was waitressing and bartending to pay rent on her tiny studio apartment in a dangerous neighborhood.

Gwen was also tough on herself. In her mind, unless she chased every carrot, tackled everything she *should* do, no matter what it did to her in the process, she would never make it to the top. And worse, she would blame herself for not being willing to do whatever it took to get there. But living this way, dragged around by the unending *shoulds* and ruled by such a harsh and unforgiving internal critic, was also painful and exhausting.

After a decade of relentlessly pushing herself, her career had basically stayed the same, but her exhaustion and dissatisfaction had grown far worse. Ten years of never saying no had left her weary, deeply disappointed, and on her way to bitter. The story she'd always told herself, that her time would come, was wearing thin and feeling less believable. Most importantly, she was growing tired of the life she was actually living—her real life, not the imaginary one that would happen later, when she was famous.

With a lot of hard work and tears, Gwen was finally able to admit to herself that she didn't want to keep struggling. She wanted a life that she would want to be living—*now*. Her present experience, her suffering, had finally become something that mattered. At last, Gwen chose to hang up her comedian's hat and enter graduate school.

The change in her was almost immediate: she felt at peace for the first time in her life. She was, as she put it, "not desperately striving to get somewhere else and to become someone more important." She even discovered that she loved puttering around the house, which in her previous incarnation, she had never allowed herself to do. Ironically, she was proud of her hard-earned ability to do nothing and for having had the courage to step off the treadmill of endless striving.

And then she met Brendon. Her new boyfriend was tall, dark, and handsome, a jet setter and a successful entrepreneur—on the fast track. Filled with ambition and talent, he (like the old Gwen) never missed an opportunity to attend an event, network, or just go the extra mile, whatever was needed to score the next deal. As she described, "Brendon's always chasing something bigger and better, and usually getting it. He's the winning version of my old self."

Soon, Gwen started talking about getting back into comedy; she started referring to her life as boring and to herself as a failure. Her coursework, which she'd described as fascinating just weeks earlier, was now pointless. The enjoyable and courageous life that she'd been so proud to claim as her own, and felt so connected to, was now average and not enough. And indeed, she experienced *herself* as just average and not enough.

Gwen had lost her connection with what her life meant to her and was now viewing and experiencing her life through the lens of what it looked like (or so she imagined) to her boyfriend. How she felt about herself was now defined by how Brendon viewed her. The respect Gwen had built for her own unique journey was gone; all that remained were a few judgments by which her jet-set partner might label her (if she wasn't too boring and average for him to even bother).

This is what we do to ourselves without even knowing we're doing it. We ignore, dismiss, and throw away our own truth, the meaning our journey holds *for us,* and we replace it with other people's stories and meaning and how our journey appears to them.

If you want to break this self-abandoning habit, you must first become aware of it, and aware of your willingness to discard your own knowing and define your life and its worth in the way other people define it. And furthermore, aware of your habit of allowing the meaning of your journey to be authored by someone else—based on what they value. Once you can see yourself doing this and see the suffering that it causes you, then you are in a position to *stop* doing it.

Playing a Character in Someone Else's Story

For six years, Naomi had been in a marriage where making love involved a few perfunctory kisses, then intercourse, and then sleep. In the day-to-day, there was no hand-holding, hugging, or as she put it, "juiciness." Naomi had been with many partners, and there was nothing she loved more than lying in bed, talking, giggling, and cuddling. She craved touch, connection, and physical intimacy. But for complicated reasons that included religion, she had married a man who was a good provider, but had little interest in physical intimacy and also seemed somewhat frightened and repelled by it. While the marriage worked in many ways, still, Naomi had always felt lonely and unsatisfied in it, making do without what she really needed.

Finally, the moment came when telling the truth wasn't so much a choice as it was a necessity; she couldn't pretend that she was okay for one more day, one more hour, or even one more minute. After years of unsuccessfully trying to stuff down and outrun her needs (she was, in fact, a marathon runner), she told the truth—out loud. She told her husband that she was lonely and felt starved for affection and closeness. She shared her deep need for more touch, physical connection, and intimacy—to be *fed* in their marriage.

Her husband's response was not what she'd hoped: she should find herself another man if she was so unhappy and dissatisfied with him. There was no point in trying to make it work because obviously he was such a big disappointment as a husband for her. But she should have known whom she married; he had never been a touchy person, so why did she think or expect that he would become that now—for her, no less? And finally: Maybe he would want to kiss her more if the house were tidier, which was what *he* craved and what *he* needed.

It seemed to Naomi that she had two options: she could either accept her husband and the marriage as it was, accept that her feelings were too dangerous to be heard, and live without the intimacy she craved, or she could leave the marriage with three small children and no income of her own, which for many reasons she didn't feel ready to do.

So she went the heartbreaking route and turned her back on herself—shut herself out of her own heart. Naomi became convinced that she was, in her words, "a first-class bitch," unfairly and overly demanding and ungrateful for her wonderful and generous man. She was a bad person for needing what her husband couldn't give and making him feel inadequate, thereby causing him to suffer. She had rejected him, which she had no right to do; her conclusion was that her needs were unfair, excessive, and invalid.

And so, Naomi did what so many of us do: she stepped right into her husband's narrative and took on the role of perpetrator in his story of victimhood. When we do this, we assume responsibility and blame for what's been defined as our illegitimate experience and undeserving needs. As the perpetrator, we accept the blame not just for having the experience we're having, but for inflicting that experience on someone else and thereby victimizing them with our truth. The solution, then, is for us to feel guilty and make up for it, do away with our damaging experience, stop trying to get what we need, and return to the business of being pleasing and having an experience that works for everyone.

If you're familiar with this mindset, your emotional fatigue may stem from the fact that you define yourself by the way other people define you. Whoever you are in their narrative is who you believe you are; however *they* experience you is how you experience yourself. And so, your energy must go into controlling, correcting, and positivizing everyone's experience of you so that you can like yourself. But in allowing your identity and self-experience to be other-defined, and letting others' storyline script your reality, you are left rudderless, without a center, and entirely untethered from yourself and your own truth. You have no choice but to feel depleted.

The Shift to Autonomy

Ironically, we are masters in figuring out and managing other people's experience, but we don't learn to discern our own experience. The idea that we could even have an experience of our own, a truth separate and free from what it means to and for everyone else, is already radical.

If you're like many women, you may never have built an autonomous relationship with yourself. And so, that's exactly what needs to happen: Start relating to yourself as someone you want to know and deeply understand. Offer your inner experience your full attention in that kind, non-judgmental, and steadfast way you do when you really care about someone. Set out to discover what's true for you, through your own eyes and heart, without everyone else's feelings, projections, and judgments in the way and mixed in. Remind yourself that you are the only one who gets to define why you do what you do, what matters to you, what's true for you, and ultimately, who you are. Starting now, claim your own story and stand in it.

The more you acknowledge and honor your own truth, the less you need anyone else to agree with or approve of it. What grows, in fact, is a need and urgency for your own approval. Taking on and trying to control other people's versions of you become less compelling and nec-essary. The key is in recognizing the ridiculousness (and tragedy) of farming out your sense of self and trying to earn external permission for your internal truth. With this key in the lock, your need to please others will transform into a need to please yourself.

Unlike what you've been taught, caring about yourself doesn't have to come at the expense of caring about others. In fact, this belief, that caring about yourself and others are mutually exclusive and you can only do one or the other, is part of the conditioning that keeps us dis-missing and rejecting our own needs. With practice, however, you will discover that you can acknowledge and honor your own experience and at the same time understand and empathize with another person's experience without either needing to be invalidated or made to be wrong. Both truths can be true, even when they're radically different and even when they conflict. As it turns out, your heart is big enough to hold all of it.

If you want to create a different kind of life, to recover from your emotional exhaustion, you have to be willing to try an unfamiliar and potentially uncomfortable path. And to walk this new path even if you're afraid and don't know where you're headed. Because if you do walk this new path, and if you stay the course, you will be actively rejecting the cultural conditioning from which you've been shaped. I promise you this: if you keep practicing this new way of relating to the world and being with yourself, the discomfort, distrust, and fear will melt away and a new clarity and strength, a new vitality, and indeed a new *you* will bloom.

When we know how to stay connected to ourselves—in our own presence while in the company of others; when we can hold onto our truth, no matter how that truth is received, judged, or rewritten, then we can let go of the beliefs and behaviors that lead to our emotional exhaustion. Once we're able to clear out the programming that's disconnected us from ourselves and drained us of our own wisdom, then we can come home to our own well of well-being.

The fact is, we women already possess our greatest source of nourishment. Lo and behold, it's us.

11

REPLENISHED: STANDING IN YOUR OWN SHOES

I started this book with a question: Why are so many women emotionally exhausted? And its natural partner: *How* can we revitalize ourselves and start getting what we really need?

You've been immersed in a powerful conditioning process, a training program in how to behave and not behave—from society, your family, education, the media, and everything else you've encountered. A process that, among other things, has taught you to manage, police, and reject your own needs. To look outside yourself for fulfillment, the answers to your deepest questions, and most of all, how to feel about yourself. All of this, in order to stay safe and belong.

You've probably faced very real threats and consequences for making yourself authentically visible and expressing your real needs. Threats that come in the form of judgments, criticism, and rejection. Like most of us, you've probably come to believe that your happiness relies on being likable, more than anything else. You may therefore have been assuming that figuring out how to make that happen—how to *be* pleasing—is the single most important self-caring action you can take for yourself. But it's not. In fact, it's this one belief, more than any other, that keeps you stuck, and emotionally exhausted in that stuckness.

Self-care, as we know it, which is sold as the answer to our exhaustion, is an insufficient remedy, ill-suited to heal what ails us. Self-care in its current iteration keeps us dependent on external sources for our internal sustenance, doubting ourselves and chasing something that will presumably give us what we need and make us better versions of ourselves. But self-care doesn't go deep or far enough; it doesn't infiltrate our emotional and spiritual marrow, and fails to address the underlying issues that create our depletion. No matter how good it smells, tastes, and feels, self-care cannot change the fact that we've abandoned ourselves in an effort to become what's wanted.

The truth is, there's no glow light, cashmere slipper, or essential oil that can persuade us to care about ourselves or make us know that we matter. None of it can connect us with our truth or establish a sense of respect and trust in our own wisdom—not in any sustainable way. We're applying an external salve to the internal condition from which we suffer and then wondering why it doesn't work, and why, after all our diligent self-care, we remain depleted and with our needs unmet.

While seemingly designed to nourish us, the current model of self-care keeps us seeking more self-care, forever on the hamster wheel—searching and spinning, and blaming ourselves. Its template is such that we are always improving, but never good enough, and never stopping to consider that we, like that dying gazelle, might already be the destination we're seeking, and the source of our own fulfillment. Giving ourselves pleasure is an important practice, and doing it without guilt is even more important, and yet we cannot entrust our deepest needs to the self-care industry, or to anyone or anything else for that matter.

Most self-help strategies provide instructions on how to behave in an empowered way, to stand up for ourselves, say *no* instead of always saying *yes*, be forthright about what we need, and ultimately, live as our *best* self. But we can't do any of these things, not in any substantial or effective way, until we can acknowledge, respect, and dignify our own truth. We can't heal our exhaustion until we can build a reverent relationship with ourselves—*all* of ourselves. And furthermore, we can't access our full vitality and power until we can trust ourselves. Our experience has to matter *to us* before we can convince anyone else that it matters. *We* have to be on our own side, to know that we're worthy of getting our needs met—that we're worthy, period—before we can *live* that knowing in the world.

In order to truly replenish ourselves, we must reprogram our fundamental conditioning. We do this by first becoming aware of it and then taking action—generating the courage to speak, walk, and embody our truth in the world—even when it means *not* being who other people would like us to be. This process demands conviction, patience, a huge supply of bravery, and self-love—for a self that hasn't yet been allowed to fully or freely live.

But here's the hard truth: if you want to discover who you are beyond all the roles you play; if you want to live as your authentic self; if you want to feel plugged into your real power and vitality, you're going to have to live without everyone else's approval and adoration. But it's well worth the effort. The fact is, you can't be on your own side and also have everyone else always on your side. Reality doesn't work that way. You have to be willing to choose yourself, choose the truth, and trust that your own support, respect, and approval are ultimately what will sustain you.

I hope that you've been absorbing this book emotionally, physically, and spiritually, and not just intellectually. I hope that you now know, in your bones, that taking care of yourself is *an inside job*, that the work happens from the inside out. And that self-care is not something you acquire. Rather, it's an attitude shift that happens in your intimate relationship with yourself. When you create an internal climate of empathy, support, and deep respect for your own truth, then you are nourishing yourself at the most fundamental level. Replenishment is in progress.

When you become more interested in how you are than how others are with you, then a new life becomes possible, necessary, and inevitable. At that point, in fact, your new life is already happening.

Grounded in your own truth, supported by your own allegiance, and empowered by your own respect—standing in your own shoes—self-care becomes something you *are* rather than something you *do*. The *you* who is caring for you is no longer separate from the *you* you're taking care of. Now you will be able to take "be good to myself" off your to-do list; the instruction simply won't make sense anymore, as it will be impossible to neglect or reject your own needs. Caring about yourself will be a given, and being good to yourself, nonnegotiable. At last, you won't need an expert (or sticky note) to tell you to do it.

Here's the good news: You don't have to live from the conditioning and false beliefs in which you've been indoctrinated. You don't have to buy into a system that convinces you that your experience and your needs are the problem, or more to the point, that *you* are the problem. Furthermore, you don't have to relate to yourself as someone who's not good enough, needs to be fixed, and is fundamentally at fault. And you don't have to keep searching for someone or something *out there* that will make you better and complete. Even though it's at the heart of everything we've been conditioned to believe, you don't have to be who others want you to be in order to get what you need and be happy. That life can be over.

Awareness is freedom: Once you can see a pattern, you can change it; you can create a different way of being, a different reality—a life that *you* design rather than one that designs you. By refusing to buy into these archaic and imprisoning beliefs, you are actively building a new self-care paradigm.

Emotional exhaustion doesn't have to be part of your story; it's not a necessary component or consequence of being female. When you practice self-care from the inside out, you will get your needs met in ways you may never have imagined. And furthermore, you will create a life that's about more than just the roles you play, being likable, and keeping yourself safe. No one tells you this, but the door to the likability cage opens *from the inside*. There is life beyond the cage, and it's more real, more dynamic, freer, and more fulfilling than anything you could live locked up inside. And indeed, the *safety* of the cage, of being liked, will transform into a new kind of safety, one that comes from being aligned with your truth. Being truthful will replace being liked as the surest way to take care of yourself.

In fact, there's no better time than now to start speaking your truth, claiming your own wisdom, and standing in your own shoes. And don't stop there...*keep* speaking your truth, *keep* claiming your own wisdom, and *keep* standing in your own shoes. It's a lifetime practice, one day at a time. With *you* firmly on your own side, you'll have the key to an infinite source of nourishment and vitality; you'll have the key to *you*. Welcome home.

ACKNOWLEDGMENTS

First, thank you, Elizabeth Hollis Hansen, for understanding my early vision for this book and supporting me along the way. Thank you, too, to Jennifer Holder, for your thoughtful input. To my dearest traveling companions, Bronwen Davis, Melissa McCool, Karen Greenberg, Anne Jablonski, Lisa Patrick, Jonathan Sachs, and Amy Belkin, thank you... for your support and friendship. Gratitude to Steve Wishnia for your steady kindness. To Jan Bronson, thank you for everything. To Frederic, thanks for the belly laughs and sound advice (which, as you know, I don't always take). Glad to have you beside me. To my girls, Juliet and Gretchen—my walking heart, I hope you will become leaders for a new generation of women who have the courage to speak their truth and to become far more than just likable. To my mom, Diane Shainberg, thank you for being such a vital life force and pointing me toward the mystery. And to my clients, thank you for teaching me every day and always opening my heart.

ENDNOTES

1.   "Stress by Gender," American Psychological Association, 2010, https://www.apa.org/news/press/releases/stress/2010/gender-stress.

2.   "Self-Care Is the Most Searched Googled Query Right Now." Times of India, May 13, 2020, https://timesofindia.indiatimes.com /life-style/health-fitness/de-stress/self-care-is-the-most-searched-google -query-right-now/articleshow/75709693.cms.

3.   "Michel Foucault: Ethics," Internet Encyclopedia of Philosophy, https://iep.utm.edu/fouc-eth/#H4.

4.   Aisha Harris, "A History of Self-Care," Slate, April 5, 2017, http://www.slate.com/articles/arts/culturebox/2017/04/the_history _of_self_care.html.

5.   Ibid.

Nancy Colier is a psychotherapist, author, interfaith minister, and public speaker. A longtime student of Eastern spirituality, she is a thought leader on mindfulness, well-being, and digital life. Featured on *Good Morning America*, in *The New York Times*, *USA Today*, and other media, Colier is also a regular blogger for *Psychology Today* and *HuffPost*. She is author of *Can't Stop Thinking*, *The Power of Off*, *Inviting a Monkey to Tea*, and *Getting Out of Your Own Way*.

Real change *is* possible

For more than forty-five years, New Harbinger has published proven-effective self-help books and pioneering workbooks to help readers of all ages and backgrounds improve mental health and well-being, and achieve lasting personal growth. In addition, our spirituality books offer profound guidance for deepening awareness and cultivating healing, self-discovery, and fulfillment.

Founded by psychologist Matthew McKay and Patrick Fanning, New Harbinger is proud to be an independent, employee-owned company. Our books reflect our core values of integrity, innovation, commitment, sustainability, compassion, and trust. Written by leaders in the field and recommended by therapists worldwide, New Harbinger books are practical, accessible, and provide real tools for real change.

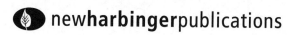 **newharbinger**publications

MORE BOOKS from
NEW HARBINGER PUBLICATIONS

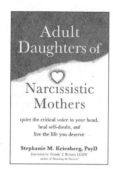
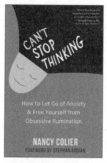
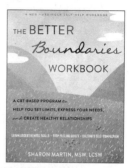
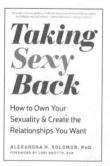
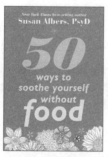
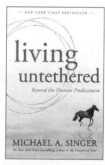

Did you know there are **free tools** you can download for this book?

Free tools are things like **worksheets, guided meditation exercises**, and **more** that will help you get the most out of your book.

You can download free tools for this book—whether you bought or borrowed it, in any format, from any source—from the New Harbinger website. All you need is a NewHarbinger.com account. Just use the URL provided in this book to view the free tools that are available for it. Then, click on the "download" button for the free tool you want, and follow the prompts that appear to log in to your NewHarbinger.com account and download the material.

You can also save the free tools for this book to your **Free Tools Library** so you can access them again anytime, just by logging in to your account! Just look for this button on the book's free tools page.

+ Save this to my free tools library

If you need help accessing or downloading free tools, visit **newharbinger.com/faq** or contact us at **customerservice@newharbinger.com**.